PRAISE FOR NAMRATA PUROHIT

'Pilates with Namrata has been life-changing for me. Not only is she motivating and superbly qualified but she is also an amazing person whose life revolves around fitness. She is now like my little sister, and we have experienced physical and mental training together that is challenging and exciting! Love her!'—Manasi Scott, singer and actress

'Namrata is a real pain to work with, and I mean that as a compliment! She's merciless and, what's worse, it comes with a smile, so you don't feel the pain until the next day. It is good pain though. She has really sorted me out'—Vishal Dadlani, artist, singer and music director

'Joining The Pilates Studio was one of the best things I've done! To work out with Namrata is so much of fun because she makes me do different things every session, and the way my body has transformed is just magical!'—Elli Avram, model and actress

'I have been doing Pilates for about five years now. When I moved to Mumbai and was looking for a Pilates instructor, I kept hearing just one name. After meeting Namrata, I quickly realized why everyone was raving about her. On the outside, she's personable, adorable and a joy to work out with. On the inside, she really knows her stuff! For someone so young, she's so accomplished in her field. And yet she's determined to keep learning more! This year, I finally got down to my ideal shape, and I can't thank Namrata enough! If you try her class just once, I can bet you'll say bye-bye to that gym membership!'—Lauren Gottlieb, actress, dancer, top scorer on *Jhalak Dikhla Jaa* (Season 6), and top-six contestant on *So You Think You Can Dance* (Season 3)

'Getting trained by Namrata is an extremely pleasing experience for the mind, and a grilling experience physically, which according to me is a great way to start the day. What's even more wonderful is that she is so young and has a long way to go in the field of fitness and Pilates'—Neha Dhupia, actress

'Training with Namrata feels like a circus act where I'm the ace acrobat! She truly works the principle of mind over body in all her workouts!'— Tanishaa Mukerji, actress

'It's been an amazing experience since I started doing Pilates; the training really makes you feel good during and after the class. You feel the muscles you never thought you had! For me, it's my favourite workout, and it feels especially great to have Namrata as my trainer—we get along really well, and I'm thankful that she has the power to make me work out hard! Also, Pilates has been helping me a lot in whatever exercises I do—it gave me more power, strength, balance. I'm really happy with the studio and my beautiful trainer!'—Izabelle Leite, actress and model

'Namrata, thank you so much for making my workout sessions fun, crisp and challenging. Not only have I seen fabulous results in toning my body, but my strength and stamina have also improved from the past! I'm extremely happy with my workouts and don't feel drained out or tired post it. Keep it going! Best wishes and loads of love, xx!'— Tina Ahuja, actress

'Namrata has made a profession out of Pilates because she follows it not just as a mode of exercise but as a lifestyle. I have learnt several aspects of correct alignment that have benefited me—not just in terms of fitness, but in life!'—Richa Chadda, actress

'Namrata's training and guidance has not only allowed me to have fun while exercising but also given me the best body I have ever had!'—Carla Dennis, model and actress

'Working with Namrata has been great. She is a young rock star, who knows how to get great results'—Abhishek Nayar, professional cricketer

'It's only been a month of training with her, but with her knowledge of Pilates, the experience has been unforgettable. Her energy and dedication is commendable. From the very first session we felt welcomed and were very comfortable to work with her. She is an amazing instructor and exhibited the exercises clearly and patiently'—Renedy Singh, professional footballer, and president, Football Players' Association of India

'Namrata is undoubtedly a wonderful Pilates trainer. She really inspires you, and that's what makes her great. After my back injury, I'm back in full form because of her!'—Bruna Abdullah, model and actress

'Thorough to the core with her work, the gifted Namrata displays a rare combination of technical finesse and youthful charm'—Suma Shirur, Olympic finalist, Arjuna Awardee and world-record holder for 10m air rifle (women)

'Namrata has taught me that you can lose weight and be fit without starving yourself. She's also taught me the importance of exercising smartly rather than killing yourself'—Hazel Keech, model and actress

'Pilates was new to me, something I had never done before. And Namrata has this amazing way of teaching exercises, which has helped me get stronger and fitter. She has helped me tone and strengthen my core muscles, giving proper balance to my body and improving my stability'—Dhawal Kulkarni, cricketer

THE
LAZY GIRL'S
GUIDE TO
BEING FIT

THE
LAZY GIRL'S
GUIDE TO
BEING FIT

NAMRATA PUROHIT

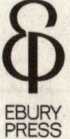

EBURY
PRESS

An imprint of Penguin Random House

EBURY PRESS

USA | Canada | UK | Ireland | Australia
New Zealand | India | South Africa | China | Singapore

Ebury Press is part of the Penguin Random House group of companies
whose addresses can be found at global.penguinrandomhouse.com

Published by Penguin Random House India Pvt. Ltd
4th Floor, Capital Tower 1, MG Road,
Gurugram 122 002, Haryana, India

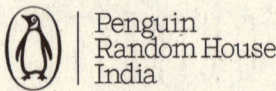

Penguin
Random House
India

First published by Random House India 2015
Published in Ebury Press by Penguin Random House India 2018

Copyright © Namrata Purohit 2015
Foreword copyright © Lisa Haydon 2015

ISBN 9788184006018

Typeset in Bembo by R. Ajith Kumar
Printed at Repro India Limited

www.penguin.co.in

MIX
Paper from
responsible sources
FSC® C047271

This is a legitimate digitally printed version of the book and therefore might not
have certain extra finishing on the cover.

*For my parents, without whom this would
never have been possible—they have made me believe in myself*

CONTENTS

FOREWORD

Let me start by saying this: Namrata is not a lazy girl. In the short time I've known her, she's asked me to go horse riding with her, which I have. Go bicycling with her, which I am yet to do. She's also whipped my ass in her Pilates class and left me groaning, 'Who knew lying down could be this exhausting?' In the last four months she's gone diving in the Andamans, been skydiving in Dubai, has been learning contemporary dance, and gone diving *again* in the Andamans. Here's what I've come to realize about this gorgeous little bohemian. Namrata is a reminder of how you want to live—reminiscent of how we all were in those bubbly teenage years when we didn't stress the small things. Only, Namrata is not a teenager any more, she just knows what's important in life and the fun bits that we should never let go of. She has all the purity and spunk of a girl who spends her time doing exactly what makes her happy: staying active and enjoying all the small joys of life.

But what stands out to me the most is the dedication and discipline it takes to live this ideal lifestyle, indulging in all the activities that take you into nature, ensuring a perfect sync between mind and body. For example, no drinking, waking up early and, not to mention, getting off one's lazy bum. All of these activities are not her way of keeping fit, necessarily. It's actually her way of having fun. Fitness is just a by-product of that.

I'm glad she started training to be a Pilates teacher so young because now it's more than just a job. Her expertise comes from intuition, from really knowing her craft for so long. Her teaching techniques are simple, intense, yet fun. Every class, I see myself doing something different and pushing myself harder. I always want to go back for more. Pursuant to a workout, I never feel dull or exhausted, instead I feel more energized and positive. Always a good day after the workout!

I constantly weigh my performance in class against hers ...

Me: *Nams, is your core always engaged throughout the day?*

Nams: *Yes.*

Me: *Even when we're riding horses?*

Nams: *Yes, especially when we are riding horses.*

So everything she does is an opportunity to engage her core? Exactly!

I discovered The Pilates Studio after running a number of marathons, which left me satisfied, but my body had taken a beating. There was a lot that needed to be fixed. Now, instead of going to the chiropractor, I go to Namrata. Pilates aligns everything, it puts your spine, hips, etc., back in the right place, and every time I walk out, I feel a sense of connection to my core through all the breathing and 'engaging' that we've spent the last hour doing. By the way, the breathing bit also feels quite meditative. It brings me right into my core, into myself. Pilates makes you aware of all your big muscles, and even the little ones you never knew existed, through simple stabilizing exercises. The first time I did Pilates, I felt silly for expending so much energy on huge strenuous repetitions at the gym, when all that was needed was the slightest focus turned inward on much more subtle movement. This reminds me of Namrata—a beautiful, little girl with huge power inside. Her carefree attitude towards life makes everything look easy—don't forget she runs the country's most successful and busy Pilates school with all manner of celebrities popping in and out all day.

On one particular day we were doing hamstring curls. Easy enough, right? Not quite. An exercise that we make a huge movement out of at the gym, with kilos of weights, gets reduced to a small movement on the Reformer (an amazing example of Pilates exercise equipment), which works all those little supporting muscles. Trust me, it's so much harder, but so much more effective.

Namrata innovates in every class, with hundreds of stabilizing exercises that kind of leave you feeling like you're playing around on the Reformer machine. It feels fun and new, like driving a new car. And no two workouts are ever the same. Namrata's observation skills are truly admirable; she's constantly correcting my form and ensuring I do each exercise correctly, so I get the most out of my workout. I have realized that it is not about doing a million but just a few repetitions correctly. Her energy in class and encouragement is amazing, leaving me with no chance of getting lazy. During our twelfth class, Nams points out during our bicycle exercise, 'I can see your hamstring.' Yep, that's what happens at The Pilates Studio.

Watch out, lazy girls. With Namrata's fitness routines, you will definitely feel energized and want to push harder and do more!

Lisa Haydon
Mumbai, 2015

INTRODUCTION

Think about it. Almost everyone you know wants that perfect body, wants to be in shape, and wants to feel healthy and strong. But only a few do something about it, while the rest give up and slowly start avoiding the topic.

I have trained all sorts of people—some who are fit and are just aiming to get fitter and stronger; some who have injuries and want to improve their strength and reduce aches and pains; sports personalities and celebrities; and some people who are not very fond of exercising and do not find enough time for it. Whoever I may be training, I believe in following one thing always, which is my ideology: Train Smart. Not everyone has the time to spend hours at the gym or on their fitness regime, and hence it is important to make the most of the limited time that we have. It is not about putting in many hours of training a week, but about making even that thirty-minute workout extremely effective. It is about using it in the most apt and fun way possible, working your body and mind smartly but thoroughly, working safely yet dynamically, ensuring a full mind-and-body workout. We all need to start sneaking in some sort of exercise and physical activity into our daily regime. This book is aimed at all the people who need some motivation and help to kick-start a regular fitness regime, and even those who believe they are doing well, but need a little change and a few fun ideas about how to get moving.

I was twelve when I started playing squash seriously. I was a late starter indeed when it came to the game. Catching up with all the other players, who had been playing since they were five or even younger, was always a challenge. As time went by, I got stronger and fitter and was slowly catching up. Just when I thought I was there, I had a terrible fall. I injured my knee—suffering an anterior cruciate ligament (ACL) injury—and had to have immediate surgery. I was sixteen at the time. This surgery is what changed my life.

After the surgery, I tried various fitness regimes to get back into form, as my squash nationals were only six months away. I was making progress, but it was slow. At the time, my father, Samir Purohit, was conducting a Pilates course in Mumbai, and he had flown down the master instructor from Canada. My father has been in the fitness field for a really long time and it seems like his passion for fitness has rubbed off on me as well. I was adamant on doing the course and seeing what Pilates was all about. I had also heard about the benefits of Pilates for rehabilitation purposes. Hoping it would help me, and also excited to learn something new, I enrolled myself for the course.

The course began and it was definitely a little difficult in the beginning. All the other people in the group had some background in fitness, plus I was the youngest one around, so it was definitely a bit intimidating for me. Since I had taken up the challenge, I had to prove to myself that I could do it, more than anyone else. I went on to successfully complete the course. I can also proudly say that my instructor was impressed. I was excited and thrilled to have succeeded. I was the youngest trained Stott Pilates instructor in the world! This was definitely a great achievement and was extremely overwhelming.

During the course, my instructor also helped me work through my knee injury, and 10 days from the start of the course, I was back to playing squash. I actually felt stronger and more balanced than I was before the surgery, which was great. It was fabulous to see the sudden improvement in my movement, stability and balance. I even felt more confident since I didn't feel that nagging pain any more. I stood fourth in the squash junior nationals that year. According to me, this was made possible, of course, thanks to my squash coach, but largely due to the wonder of Pilates.

The sheer magic of Pilates is what made me think that people here in India were really missing out on this amazing form of exercise. The exercise is not strenuous, it is injury-free and, most importantly, is very time-efficient. It is amazing to see all that Pilates can achieve—it is great for strength, flexibility, endurance, balance, stability, confidence, movement and improving lean body mass—the list can go on and on. Also, the beauty of this form is that anybody can do it, from a 10-year-old to an 80-year-old, a fitness freak or a lazy person, a sportsperson, dancers, people with special conditions—anybody! And it will do wonders for each and every person. This is when my father and I decided to open The Pilates Studio in Mumbai.

In the past six years spent training various people, I have only become more and more convinced by the importance of being fit. Some people I have trained have had injuries, while others have been extremely fit and have wanted to try something new. The most fun transformation, though, is that of a person who comes to me not liking to work out at all, to one who just cannot stop exercising. This is the metamorphosis I am hoping to achieve in each and every one of you. Let's make this the start to a great journey, as fitness and exercise are great addictions to have.

I believe it is never too late to start—even starting slow and small is fine. All we have to do is find something we enjoy and stick to it. Most of us do not realize the importance of exercising when we are young. Many people have naturally thin bodies and hence believe that they do not need to work out. Exercising, though, is not only about looking good, it is about feeling good, feeling energized and being healthy inside out. Fitness is much broader than just what the body appears to be. And merely being thin does not mean you are fit. And for anybody who thinks that they have reached a point of no return, trust me, it is never too late. Just don't be lazy. Get started now—not tomorrow! The problem is that the lazier you are, the lazier you get; therefore, a good time to start is now. Don't wait for tomorrow, don't wait another day! Just get started and enjoy the benefits of exercising. Find a regime that works for you, a regime you enjoy, and you will never want to stop. It is somewhat addictive. Once you start and see the benefits and the difference in the way you feel and look, you will not want to stop.

The reason I am writing this book is especially to connect with young girls. Being in the same phase of life as them, I do understand what we want and what we need. I hope this book helps girls get up, get out and get FIT!

1

POTATO, POTAATO: DECONSTRUCTING THE COUCH–POTATO SYNDROME

A couch potato. Is that you? Do you watch a lot of TV? Do you play a lot of video games? Do you often have *The Vampire Diaries/Gossip Girl* marathons? Do you love being on the computer? Or do you simply enjoy sitting and doing nothing? If your answer to any of these questions is yes, then a couch potato is what you might be! Don't worry, it's not as bad as it sounds. By the end of this book, you will be up and about.

We all pass through a phase where we want to do absolutely nothing. We just want to sit endlessly and aimlessly in one place, enjoying the feeling of doing nothing, watching television, playing on the computer, or sitting at the desk and working. For a little time this may seem all right, but soon you start to realize that you are becoming lazier and lazier each day. Even getting your own glass of water might start seeming a nuisance. Well, the truth is that sitting and being lazy will only make you lazier as each day passes. So the right time to get up and get out is *now*!

So what exactly is a couch potato? The couch-potato syndrome, in the typical sense, is when you spend hours in front of a television or computer, with barely any activity. These days most of us spend hours sitting. We sit and watch TV, play on the computer, sit in class, sit at work, sit in a car—all we seem to do is just *sit*. Many studies have proven that there is a strong link between watching television and obesity. Most of the day we are sitting, slouched over, in all sorts of awkward positions. Various research has shown that sitting for hours could be very harmful and lead to a large number of problems in the long run. One major and obvious problem is that sitting for hours leads to bad posture. We see many people with rounded shoulders who are always slouching and whose heads tend to be bent forward. This is the typical posture of a person who spends a lot of time watching TV or being on the computer. Bad posture may not seem like such a big problem initially, but it is known to be a window to various other problems, aches and pains. Sitting for hours can increase inflammation in the body, which can cause heart problems. Sitting for hours can also make you feel blue and depressed. It can increase the chances of diabetes and cancer. But the most obvious and visible outcome of sitting for hours is obesity.

Obesity is a condition in which the body stores excess fat; this excess fat has various negative effects. Obesity can cause heart diseases, arthritis, osteoporosis and Type 2 diabetes, amongst other things. No, I am not trying to scare you, but this is all true. I believe that every problem has a solution, so start now and save yourself all the trouble later. Why wait another day and make it tougher and tougher to get fit and back in shape? The most effective way to treat obesity is to follow a healthy diet and a fitness regime. A diet should be healthy, and no drastic changes should be made in the food intake. A fitness regime should be gradual, and one should not overexert oneself. In the next few chapters, we will talk about introducing exercises slowly and safely into your daily regime. Let's tackle obesity and the problems related to it— now rather than later—and start following and incorporating a healthy lifestyle. It's all about 'Training Smart'. There are many reasons obesity is such a problem in today's day and age; it is only going to get worse as we grow older and witness further growth in technology and more pressure at work. These issues need to be tackled by introducing exercise as a compulsory part of our daily living.

Have you ever wondered why they say that schooldays are the best days of your life? Many people believe it is because children face less pressure; but this, according to me, is not entirely true. Children are under pressure to get good grades and submit assignments on time; they are also subject to peer pressure and the pressure to perform well in co-curricular activities. We all had responsibilities and assignments even when we were young. The one thing that was different in our schooldays was that we spent a lot of time running about, playing games, learning a sport or to swim and skate. Those were the days we went out of the house and into the neighbourhood, played hide-and-seek with our friends, and kept moving and enjoying ourselves. Many schools had a compulsory games period, when you had to play some game for an hour. Some schools also made it compulsory to learn how to swim and took the students swimming once a week. For example, my school had a swimming class for one and a half hours every week; we also had a games period one hour every week in which we learned how to play football, handball, basketball, hockey and kabbadi; then we had co-curricular activities that involved dramatics, which also kept us moving; we had a utility period when we all enrolled for different activities that interested us such as cookery, pottery, aerobics, etc.; and last but not least, we had a 45-minute yoga class every week. This helped our minds relax and de-stress. I can proudly say that anyone who has ever been a part of my school knows how to swim and how to play at least one or two sports properly. I didn't realize then, but thinking about it now, all of it was a great workout. We didn't realize back then, the importance of all those activities, we just had fun doing them. Now at a later stage in life, when we have to reintroduce those physical activities compulsorily, we understand why playing was made compulsory at such a young age. Not only did it help us stay fit and active but it also relaxed us and helped us forget all our other pressures. After this we would be energized and it would be easier to concentrate during lectures and focus on what we had to do and complete assignments and homework without feeling too pressurized about it. What people say about schooldays being the best days of one's life is true. And I believe it is largely due to the amount we played and moved around which helped us relax, de-stress and have fun. This itself proves the importance of staying active.

As we grow older, we start focusing more on our work, academics and our careers, and outdoor activities are mostly abandoned. This is when we start getting lethargic and lazy. This is the stage in our life when we need to introduce exercise as a compulsory part of our daily regime. This will not only help us maintain our weight and health but will also increase concentration levels and help us focus better.

Another problem is the growth of technology in today's day and age. In the old days, when there was no television and video games, obesity was rare among youngsters. It was associated more with lethargic older people. Unfortunately, however, lethargy is very common among kids, teenagers and young adults today. Children no longer play outdoors; most want to stay at home and play games on the computer or on the PlayStation. Most plans that youngsters make revolve around going out to dinner, watching a movie or coming home and playing on the Xbox or PlayStation, while others are busy looking for a job or working 10–12 hours a day. Teenagers rarely make plans to play football or cricket, go cycling, jogging, or simply take a walk.

Technology has taken over our lives. These days, people are less active because technology has made our lives easier. Almost everything can be done with the help of machines. For example, people no longer need to wash their own clothes or dishes because of the existence of washing machines and dishwashers. We use vehicles for even the shortest journeys, which means we are sitting most of the time. Manual-labour requirements have decreased, and most jobs are desk jobs and thus sedentary in nature. All this has led to a decrease in the amount of physical activity we undertake.

It would be unfair on my part to blame this lack of activity only on the amazing growth in technology—it is also due to academic and work pressure. The pressure on young adults to achieve more and more is tremendous. Writing endless examinations coupled with the pressure to excel, carrying out assignments and projects, research work and internships, as well as the pressure of succeeding in extracurricular activities, have grown in the past few decades. This has left us with less time. It feels as though the day has fewer hours than before. I know we are under a lot of pressure to achieve success in every sphere, but if we really want to do something, we can do it. I am a strong believer in time management—if you want to do something, you will always be able to find the time for it.

Let me give you my own example—and also show off just a tiny bit. I majored in economics, which meant I had a lot to study. I took part in college competitions and activities. I simultaneously ran The Pilates Studio and trained various people. I also managed to make time for horse riding and squash, twice a week; because of my great love for the two sports, I'd wake up at 6 a.m. to pursue them. I love dancing, so I squeezed in dance classes, 4 days a week, and also found time to practise Pilates on my own. Time management is the key, my friends. If your desire to achieve something is strong, you will find a way to achieve it. As for finding the time to work out, all you need is about 30 minutes a day to keep your body active. These 30 minutes can be found at the start of your day, during your lunch break, or even when you get home. Once you start enjoying these 30-minute workouts and they become part of your regular routine, you will find time to make it a 40-minute workout. Just find a routine you enjoy, and you will be able stick to it. Also, once you start seeing the difference in your body and your skin, and the increase in your energy levels, you will want to work out more. If you want it, you can do it! Besides, your body and mind need it, so you should find the time!

It's not only about the way you may end up looking, but being a couch potato is very harmful for other reasons too. Being a couch potato and spending hours sitting can cause severe back pain and lead to bad posture and also an increased risk of heart diseases, diabetes and arthritis. Being lazy also slows down your metabolic rate, which increases your fat percentage: you will have little or no strength, and your energy levels will keep dropping. The basic logic is that the lazier you are, the lazier you will get. Do not reach a stage where you have to compulsorily find time to work out due to injuries, aches and pains, or ill health. Start now, so that you can avoid all the pain and trauma to your body at a later date, and just enjoy having a fabulous body, lots of energy and true health. Get up and move *now*!

We tend to make a million excuses as to why we can't work out on a certain day. Today, you may decide you will start your workout tomorrow, tomorrow you may have to finish the project you are supposed to submit the day after, and the day after, you are so tired from the project work of the previous day that you will have to start your workout 'tomorrow' again. Something or the other always comes up— sometimes we tend to convince ourselves that today is not a good day to start as we have to go out at night; or tomorrow might be a long day at work, so we should not exercise to avoid a sore body; or today, that our head is hurting, so we will start tomorrow. Do not find an excuse to skip the workout! Working out is not only about your body or looking good, it's more than just that.

Working out regularly is a way of life. It is about feeling great. Your mind will be more active and you will feel more positive. When you exercise, your body releases chemicals called endorphins, which trigger a positive feeling. Due to the release of endorphins, exercise has been proven to improve self-esteem, reduce stress, improve sleep and lessen feelings of anxiety and depression. Exercising is a must, and a good exercise routine will not decrease your energy levels but actually increase them. It will elevate your mood and make working and focusing on your daily tasks easier. An exercise routine that leaves you mentally and physically drained is not ideal—you should feel active mentally and feel great physically after a good workout.

In April 2012, I had a client walk into my studio with her father. She wasn't really fat, but she wasn't feeling good about herself either. She came in, and we immediately noticed the rounded shoulders, the slouching and the lazy dragging-your-feet walk. Her father unhappily told us that his daughter had never worked out in her life, was very lazy and often felt blue. She was only nineteen years old then. She was not confident about herself or the way she looked. She was also a bit anxious about working out, but due to her persuasive father she had decided to join the studio and give Pilates a shot.

In her first class, my client was slow and not very pleased about having to work out, but because she had enrolled for 12 sessions and due to her father's determination to get her fit, she had to come in regularly. In her first class, she did not understand most of the exercises and went through the routine slowly. I went along with her; I understood her strength levels and did not overdo any exercise, and so the workout was not very difficult, and was better than nothing. Another 3 sessions went by where we were just building on what we had done in the first class, little by little. The aim was to gradually get my client's confidence up, relax her, and make her understand the movements and their importance. For the fourth session, my client walked in with a smile—it was the very first time she had done so. Her shoulders were—not to my surprise—consciously held back in place, and to my pride, she had subconsciously begun walking without dragging her feet. She told me she felt good and was ready for the workout. This simple change in attitude is what working out can do—my client, in just four sessions, had stated that she felt happier and that she had more energy. That was the change I had been looking forward to. I was looking not only for a change in weight but also a change in attitude towards the workout—the energy-level increase was what I was excited about, and the better posture was what was important.

On completion of her twelfth session, my client decided to sign up for the next three months. We continue to work together even today. She has lost a lot of weight and is now fit and strong. She loves her workouts and doesn't miss a single class. She feels energized after a workout and feels more positive. Instead of feeling drained after her workout, she is ready to face the challenges of the day and feels fresh and active. Her concentration levels have increased, her patience and determination has improved and, of course, most of all she loves her body and is confident about herself. Even when she is travelling, she finds a way to stay active; she does 15-minute workouts in her room at the hotel, but she never misses a workout. This is really what working out does to you; it is somewhat addictive once you find a routine you like. It is a great addiction to have. My client is just one example amongst the million people who have found a positive change in their lives once they have begun to work out.

Each day you postpone starting a workout regime, it gets harder to work out the next day. The more you sit in your bed or laze around, the harder it gets to push and motivate yourself to get up and move for a workout. Moving around and staying active should be a major part of your life. It's not just about adding exercise to your daily routine—which is very important—but also doing simple daily chores yourself. Get up and fetch your own glass of water. If you have to talk on the phone, try walking around and talking. Instead of making an intercom call, go personally and see your co-workers. Doing all these simple things will keep you moving. Even if you are sitting during a lecture, get up and move about in the short breaks between classes. If you are working, be aware that it's important to get up and take a small walk every 30–40 minutes. Try not to sit for long stretches, because sitting continuously is very harmful. Keep moving—that is the key.

BEING THIN DOESN'T MEAN BEING FIT

A common misunderstanding is that being thin means being fit. Having a thin body is quite different from having a fit body. I hear this line frequently: 'She is thin, she does not need to work out.' Unfortunately or fortunately, exercising is not just for those people who want to lose weight but for everyone. Everybody needs exercise in some form or the other. A thin person may have a different regime from someone a little fatter, but that does not mean that the thin person does not need to work out. When you are fit, you feel and look strong, you have more energy and you love yourself for what you are. Fitness is a lot more than what your body looks like. When you set your fitness goal, it is important to think about getting fitter and not thinner. Remember to work your body from the inside out. Don't just think about lifting heavier weights, know your strengths and weaknesses, and work hard towards making your weaknesses your strengths. In case of injuries and aches and pains, first take care of them. Strengthen the muscles around them, and correct your posture and any imbalances. Start slow. Don't jump right into a crazy fitness regime, as this will do more harm than good. It is important to increase your stamina and strength gradually—it cannot be done overnight. Fitness is about having stamina and endurance, and being strong, flexible, energetic and injury-free. Being fit and working out will also make you more positive, help you concentrate better and relax. Fitness is about the development of the mind and the body—it's the connection between mind and body. It's a complete state of well-being.

Do not get influenced by trends or what others are doing. Every day there is some new trend; one day the trend is being size zero, the next day seems to be all about flaunting curves. You cannot possibly put your body through all that. Drastic changes and fluctuations are not good for your body. Set a specific goal that best suits you and your body type and stick to it. You know your body, you know what looks best on you. Don't pressurize yourself by trying to adopt the trends going around. A lot of times you wake up in the morning and read a newspaper with an ad that claims so-and-so got a perfect body in 4 weeks, which will make you wonder why you can't achieve the same. Give yourself enough time. This is not a race! Do not feel disheartened when you hear stories about people getting in shape and getting six-pack abs in 4 weeks. You will reach your ultimate goal and get your desired body, but you have to be patient and stick to your regime, and you will get there. Eat healthy, work out well, do it right, and you will get there the correct way and be able to maintain it as well. You know what's best for you. Besides, if you have the curves, I'd say flaunt. If you have it, flaunt it!

It is extremely important to know your body well. All of us have different body types. Some are naturally thin, while others are curvy. Each person's body structure is different. It is extremely important to love your body for what it is and give it your best. As they say, your body is your only permanent home. Love it for what it is and take care of it. Whatever your body structure, make it the best it can be. The different body types are:

❖ **The Hourglass Shape:** The hips and the bust are approximately the same size, while the waist is narrow.

❖ **The Pear Shape:** The hip measurement is more than the bust measurement, with a narrow waist.

❖ **The Broccoli Shape:** The bust is the widest part, while the waist and the hip are almost the same.

❖ **The Apple Shape:** The shoulders are broad and the hips narrow.

Whatever your body type, exercising is important. Enhance the different parts of your body and add more shape to it by getting a good workout. Tone your arms and legs, and make your waistline look even better. You can always work towards a better body. Tone and strengthen each muscle in your body. No body type is bad; no matter what your body type is, you can make it look great. Tone all the muscles in your body and shape them to your structure, and you are all set. There is no limit to how fit you can become. Every day you can have a new goal, every day a new target. You have got to keep trying, got to keep pushing yourself to go that one step further.

Remember: You need to keep moving, and get off the couch. Even if it's just walking, you're still doing more than the person sitting on a couch. Any sort of movement will burn calories, but sitting on the couch will not. There are so many different fitness regimes that you can do: dancing, Pilates, yoga, horse riding, going to the gym, etc. There are many options, and finding one you enjoy is not very difficult. What you must remember is that training and a fitness regime do not involve spending hours at the gym every single day. Short, intense sessions are ideal to achieve a great body. Training every day for hours will not get you better results; in fact, it will reduce the quality of your physique due to over-training. Working out 3–4 times per week is all you need to get fit. Four hours out of the typical 168-hour week, that's it! Of course, this should be accompanied by a good nutritional plan. Now, it doesn't sound all that hard, does it?

2

KICK: INSPIRE YOURSELF

What have you always wanted to do? Here are some inspirational ideas to motivate you. Let's start with some motivational quotes I love, which may inspire you to go for it as well:

- ❖ 'Every time you stay out late, every time you sleep in, every time you miss a workout, every time you don't give your 100 per cent, you make it that much easier for me to beat you'—Unknown

- ❖ 'You can have results, or you can have your excuses. You cannot have both'—Unknown

- ❖ 'Make the most of yourself . . . for that is all there is of you'—Ralph Waldo Emerson, American poet, philosopher and essayist

- ❖ 'Pain is temporary. It may last a minute, or an hour, or a day, or a year, but eventually it will subside and something else will take its place. If I quit, however, it lasts forever'—Lance Armstrong, former American professional road-racing cyclist

❖ 'Mental will is a muscle that needs exercise, just like the muscles of the body'—Lynn Jennings, retired American long-distance runner

❖ 'How am I to know what I can achieve if I quit?'—Jason Bishop

❖ 'There are only two options regarding commitment: You're either in or you're out. There's no such thing as life in between'—Unknown

❖ 'Success must be felt within before it can be seen on the outside'—Unknown

❖ 'There are plenty of difficult obstacles in your path. Don't allow yourself to become one of them'—Ralph Marston, writer and publisher of The Daily Motivator.

❖ 'The act of taking the first step is what separates the winners from the losers'—Brian Tracy, professional speaker and author

❖ 'Great souls have wills; feeble ones have only wishes'—Chinese proverb

❖ 'Make sure your worst enemy doesn't live between your own two ears'—Laird Hamilton, champion surfer

❖ 'If you just get out of your own way . . . it's amazing what will come to you'—Laird Hamilton, champion surfer

❖ 'Being exhausted is in your mind. Push through and you will be surprised how much more you can actually do'—Yours truly

❖ 'The pain is just weakness leaving your body!'—Unknown

❖ 'Achieving your goal can be as easy as you want it to be. Regular work pays'—Yours truly

❖ 'No one can push you the way you push yourself'—Yours truly

❖ 'I'll do it tomorrow = I'll never do it'—Yours truly

❖ 'Create your own deadlines! Don't rely on someone else's!'—Yours truly

❖ 'Break me physically, but you will never break me mentally'—Yours truly

Now that you have absorbed these quotes, you should already feel more inclined towards starting your workout! Let me try and help you some more.

Making excuses to avoid exercising is not going to get you anywhere. Saying that you have no time to exercise is not true—you can find the time if you really want to. Out of the 24 hours in a day, all you need is 30 minutes to get a decent exercise regime going and get you moving on the road to fitness. Stop being lazy as this will get you nowhere. Putting on excessive weight is not the only harmful effect of being lazy; you will tend to feel blue, have less energy, and will slowly start to feel bad about yourself. This can easily be avoided by exercises and keeping yourself active. Regular physical activity is one of the best things you can do for yourself.

We all find time to eat, sleep or go out with friends. Similarly, we must find time to work out. You do not need many hours every day for this; you can start with small, basic exercises that keep you moving and also burn a lot of calories. Even exercising 15–20 minutes at home, to start with, is great. Well, doing something is better than nothing, isn't it? And as they say, even a slow walk means you are doing better than the person on the couch. So do it!

If you don't find time for your body now, you will have to find time for it later. What I mean to say is that if you don't take care of yourself now and exercise, you will have to find time later when health issues creep up. Don't wait to reach that stage to start an exercise regime as that is not a happy state to be in. You may be injured or have other health problems, which could have easily been avoided by regular physical activity. So do your best to avoid the stress, and stay fit all through your life.

Exercising doesn't only mean going to the gym and lifting weights; you can also do some exercises at home or other fun activities that burn calories. Find something you enjoy, something that interests you—there is always that one regime that will work best for you. Keep trying new things until you find something you enjoy and then stick to it. You can even do different activities every day or every week. Join a dance class that you can go to once or twice a week, go play a sport on another day, the next day work out at home and, sometimes, just go to your local park or promenade and walk. This will keep things interesting, and getting bored of doing the same thing all the time will be out of question.

Let me list out a few critical reasons why you should exercise:

❖ **Weight Loss:** Most people's primary motivation to exercise is to lose weight. Many a time, the only reason people want to exercise is to lose weight and look slim and fit. Although, in my personal opinion, this is not the only reason you should exercise, it is an important one nonetheless. It is not only about the way you look with the increased weight—this is only a matter of perception—but it is the problems and health hazards that additional weight carries with it. Exercising can prevent weight gain. When you exercise you burn calories and therefore lose weight.

❖ **Improves the Mood and Helps to De-stress:** Exercise, and you will feel good. Exercising helps you relax and takes your mind off stressful things. It also makes you feel great about yourself. Due to the release of endorphins, exercising helps you feel positive. I assure you that once you start exercising regularly, you will start feeling much better and will be happier with yourself.

❖ **Energizes:** Exercising will give you an ample amount of energy. You will start feeling more energized throughout your day. Since exercise increases muscle strength and endurance, you will have more energy to take you through the day's activities. It also makes your cardiovascular system work more efficiently.

❖ **Improves Health:** In general, exercising will make you a healthier person. It improves your sleep, keeps your weight in check and, can, among other things, help prevent arthritis, depression and strokes.

❖ **Exercising Is Actually Fun:** Contrary to what most people think, exercising is not boring. Going to the gym is not the only way to exercise. You can find an activity that interests you, as now there are various options available. And even if you do start going to the gym, you can make it fun there too. Exercising is addictive, and it is a good addiction to have. Start doing it and see the results—you won't want to stop.

❖ **Helps You Sleep Better:** Exercising will help you get better sleep. You will be able to sleep faster and deeper. Just ensure you do not exercise too close to your bedtime as it could be counterproductive and energize you.

❖ **Helps Reduce Anxiety:** Doing some moderate-to-high-intensity exercises can help you calm down.

❖ **Helps Get More Done:** Due to the energy and freshness that exercising gives you, you will be able to focus more and get more work done. Studies have shown that working people who exercise tend to be more productive than those who don't.

Now that you know some of the most basic benefits of exercising, you should want to reap those benefits and start your regime today! Especially because it is not too hard to maintain a healthy lifestyle as it is definitely not time-consuming.

Remember that you are not in competition with the world, but with yourself. You have to motivate yourself and push yourself enough. No one can push you beyond a point, hence self-motivation is extremely important. You have to want to be better than you were the day before.

How to Motivate Yourself

The best way to stay motivated is to set a realistic and time-bound goal. Setting goals that are overambitious and unreasonable will only lead to disappointments. Set a goal that you know you are capable of achieving, but which is hard enough to push you. For example, if you can do 5 push-ups properly, do not set an unreasonable goal of doing 50 push-ups after 5 days, but a reasonable one, like 10 push-ups after 5 days. If A is the easiest goal to achieve, B is a little difficult but achievable with some dedication, and C is very difficult—choose B. Choose the middle path. Do not make it too easy or too difficult for yourself. Any goal should be SMART—Simple, Measurable, Achievable, Reasonable and Time-bound.

Another important thing to do is look at your image in the mirror. Ask yourself if that is really what you want to look like. You will know what looks great and what doesn't. You will know from where you need to lose weight. Once you know what your problem areas are, work towards making those areas of your body your assets. We all want that perfect bikini body, so look in the mirror, check yourself out, and decide how you are going to go about achieving that body.

Try on any of the old clothes you may have kept. Have they become tight for you? Then maybe it's time to exercise and get back into them!

Another great thing to do is to get a dress that you absolutely love, but in a smaller size. This will motivate you to push yourself and work harder to get into that dress in the shortest possible time.

Sometimes, what also helps is putting up a picture in your room, or as the display picture on your phone, of someone fit, to inspire you to fight to get into shape. Every time you see that picture, you will want to get there, you will not want to eat that packet of chips and you will feel super guilty every time you eat that butter popcorn.

You could also put up a picture of yourself in your room of when you were once fit or of the body you would like to get back to. This will remind you that you too can be fit and that you too were slim at one point. You just need to get up and get out and you can be back to your ideal weight.

A lot of people think that they have reached a point of no return and, hence, do not care any more. Always remember that it is never too late to start. You can get back in shape at any time and at any age. You may need to be patient, yes. It may take some time, but with some perseverance you can achieve that ultimate level of fitness. So don't let anything disappoint you or keep you from working out. If you are conscious about going to the gym because of your weight, start with exercising in the comfort and privacy of your own home. This too can help and will make you feel stronger and better. Once you gain some confidence, take the journey outside: go for walks, cycle, jog. Remember that beauty is in the eye of the beholder—just because you may be overweight does not make you less pretty than anyone else. You know you are beautiful and you need to love yourself before anybody else can. If you are confident, if you are ready to work towards getting fitter, what anyone else thinks does not matter. And if the people at the gym are too busy judging you, well, remember that they are not getting their workout done. You need to ensure that you stay focused and do your workout. What anyone else does or thinks really does not matter.

The popular saying 'No pain, no gain' is one that often keeps people away from fitness regimes. Don't feel disheartened by this. When you exercise, it is natural for your body to get tired, but this does not mean that you will experience pain. Pain is your body's way of telling you that something is wrong. Pain is just 'painful', but trust me, exercising is not. The exercises you do tire your muscles, but they do not hurt your muscles. I often use the term 'good pain'. There is a big difference between the 'good' pain of an exercise and bad pain. Good pain is really not painful—it's just your muscles telling you that you are tired. Doing an exercise until your muscles reach a point of fatigue is fine, and as soon as you reach this point, you must stop. If you are exercising correctly, you will not feel any bad pain. Soon, you will start enjoying the good pain that exercise gives you. Savour every moment of it.

Ask yourself a few questions to assess your fitness:

❖ Do you feel energized?
❖ Can you touch your toes while keeping your knees straight?
❖ Do you breathe deeply?
❖ Do you sleep well at night?
❖ Can you climb 5 floors without becoming highly breathless?
❖ Can you do at least 5 push-ups?
❖ Can you do 20 squats without getting tired?

❖ Can you do a 100-metre sprint without being unreasonably tired?
❖ Can you jog 400 metres non-stop?

These are a few questions you need to ask yourself. If even one of your responses is *no*, that means it is time to work out and get fit. In a short period of time, the answers to these questions should change to *yes*. These are basic things you should be able to do. It is not that difficult, and if you work out regularly, you will be able to achieve most of it in less than a month.

Another important aspect of your fitness regime is finding a good trainer who can push you and motivate you. Your trainer should know your strengths and weaknesses, and customize the workout as per your needs. The workout your trainer gives you should be safe and simple—but smart. As I always say, follow the KISSS—yes, 'kiss' with an additional 's', if I may—principle: Keep It Safe, Simple and Smart. Your workout should not cause any injuries, and the pace and strength of the workout should increase gradually. You should always feel challenged but never demotivated by not being able to do something. You should feel pushed, but not overworked. Trust yourself. You know your body, so when you do start a regular regime with your trainer, you will know when you are doing too much. Always keep your trainer informed about your goals, the reason you are working out, and any injuries or health conditions.

There is no age limit to stop staying healthy. My grandmother—who, I must add, is absolutely stunning—is still active and very healthy and strong. She is the most beautiful lady I know, and definitely one of the most active for her age. She is the light that keeps my family going, and her positive aura is a permanent motivator. She is probably more active than most teenagers and twenty-somethings. She wakes up early, does a little bit of yoga and eats healthy. My Nani has taken up her hobby as her profession. She loves plants and gardening and has hence started her own nursery. She is outdoors almost every day, getting orders ready and taking care of her own plants. Spending time outdoors is extremely good for health. Even after all this, she still has the energy to go for an evening walk. She also cooks for us often and makes all my favourite dishes. She even came for our Pilates classes when we held them close to her house.

Nani knows the importance of staying healthy and active, and enjoys every moment. She refuses to rest, which is good, as staying active is extremely important, but of course she also ensures she gets adequate amounts of sleep. You can never keep her away from her work and her exercise. Her diet is also extremely admirable. She makes the most delicious mohanthal (a sumptuous Rajasthani dessert), but is satisfied with only a bite—a quality I wish I had. She eats all the necessary vegetables and fruit she needs to every day. Her overall lifestyle is what we must try to achieve. It is a balanced way of living. Due to her balanced lifestyle, she has energy, is always happy and spreading happiness, is fit and active, and is someone from whom we should learn and take inspiration from. Waking up early, doing some exercise, going outdoors, meeting her friends regularly and eating super healthy—this is what all of us need in our lives.

I will give you another example of someone we all know.

Bruna Abdullah, the beautiful, bubbly actor, did not like working out. She had tried the gym and it was definitely something she did not enjoy. She thought this was the only option at that point and, disappointed, she stopped working out. During this phase she unfortunately suffered from a bad injury: a slipped disc.

What is a slipped disc? The spinal column is made up of 26 vertebrae that are cushioned by discs. These discs absorb shock from activities such as walking, running and lifting weights, and so protect the bones in this manner. A disc has two parts to it: the inner portion and the tough outer-portion. In case of an injury, the inner portion of the disc tends to protrude through the outer portion. This is what a slipped disc is. It may happen in any part of the spine.

Bruna had a slipped disc in her lower back. Being a performer, she had to recover her health fast. She had no choice but to work out. She tried the gym, but it did not seem to help her much. After two years of struggling with her injury and fighting through the pain, she had had enough. This is when she met a physiotherapist who suggested that she come to me and try Pilates. Knowing her condition, I started her off on the Reformer (a Pilates exercise machine), and got her moving and understanding movement. We worked slowly and steadily, focusing on rebuilding her confidence. Only four sessions through, and Bruna came back to me, saying she had no more pain. She was taken aback at her sudden improvement and fell in love with Pilates. She hasn't felt the pain since, and has been regularly dancing and performing. As I keep saying, this is all the magic of Pilates.

Bruna realized the importance of being fit and has not

looked back since. She loves working out now and is regular with it. She also understood that being fit does not mean being skinny, it is about feeling good, being strong, having enough energy and preventing injury. She had a slipped disc, but it is exercise that got rid of her pain. You have to find the correct form of exercise for yourself and work accordingly. Nothing should stop you from following a good fitness regime, and that is exactly what Bruna is doing.

Bruna did Pilates 2–3 times a week for an hour. During her sessions, she was focused and determined to get fit and strong. We ensured that we strengthened her glutes and core to decrease the pressure and pain she felt in her back. Her core got stronger and stronger with each session. We started with simple exercises, slowly progressing to more complicated and challenging ones. Bruna initially did Pilates-mat work and Reformer-based work, progressing to using the Cadillac and the Ladder Barrel (other Pilates equipment). Every workout Bruna does is different, challenging and fun. The lovely thing about her is that she understands the importance of fitness and does everything she is told. She does not cheat during her routine, and I know that even if for some reason I am not watching she will always complete what she has to do. She is a very good Pilates girl and has imbibed the importance of the Pilates principle. We all love her at the studio as she has great positive energy and is always smiling.

This example basically proves that no matter what, you must exercise. Obviously, if you have an injury, you must take your doctor's permission before you start a fitness regime.

Different people do different forms of exercise. Something that might be fun for one person might be extremely boring for someone else. For example, I know someone who has a stationary bike at home and just cycles on that to stay fit. She enjoys it as she can read her favourite books while working out, and can even watch TV if she wants to. There is another friend of mine who, if I asked her to cycle at home, would definitely think I had gone mad. She loves going outdoors, and cycles in parks and on promenades, enjoying the breeze and fresh air. Similarly, what you like might be completely different, and that is fine, but you just have to do it.

Something else that also really helps is finding a workout buddy. This will help you whenever you are feeling lazy, because your workout buddy will then push you and force you to get out, expecting the same in return. I would say, find someone who is almost at the same fitness level as you, so that you can do things together, plan a proper routine and work together. You will not want to see them do better than you, and therefore you will challenge yourself to try and stay ahead of the game. This way, you will always do more than you expect, and both your workout buddy and you will get fit and achieve your goals. Jogging, strength-training and any other form of exercise is great to do with someone as you will want to run faster, or at least try and keep up, lift more—and push harder. You should just want to go for it, and whenever you feel you are slowing down, your buddy will always be there to push you.

Whenever you feel lazy about that 40-minute workout, just tell yourself that you will run for only 10 minutes. Inevitably, you will feel energized and will actually complete the 40-minute workout. There are so many people out there to inspire and motivate us. Seeing some before-and-after pictures could actually work for you. Yes, it is possible to lose that much weight—perhaps not in an unrealistic time frame—but given enough time, and if you work out the correct way, you will lose the weight.

Anybody and everybody can exercise and find something that works for them. Look around you—there will be something you like, there has to be. As rightly said by someone wise, 'Every journey begins with a single step.' So, to start your journey to complete fitness, you need to take the first step, and in most cases, it is just a step off your couch, to start with. You can't keep waiting for the perfect moment to start, a specific occasion or day, as that will never happen! You've got to start now. There is no better time than now.

Remember that yesterday was the day you said you would start tomorrow, and that tomorrow is today, so you must start now. What you are doing now, your fitness regime, is for you, not for your mom, not for your dad, not for your dog or your best friend, and definitely not for me—it is for you. It is what you deserve to give yourself. Your mind and body deserve to get what they need, and you owe it to yourself to fulfil those needs. Keep pushing, keep pushing, you never know how much further you can go if you just push yourself. Just don't give up. If you fall down, start over. If you're tired, fight it; take a short break and go for it. Exercising is a way of life. It is how you should be living.

3

CAT: MOVEMENT AND
STRETCHES

I cannot emphasize enough the importance of movement and stretching in our lives. What exactly do I mean by *movement*? It means, in simple words, *changing a position*. That may just mean lifting your arm or changing the position of your legs. Any form of physical activity involves movement. Lifting weights, walking, skipping and playing football all involve movement of the body.

Human beings were built to move and, in the earlier ages, movement was a regular part of a person's life. In a society that was primarily agrarian, people moved all the time. They spent the day doing one activity after another. They were always on their feet, working and moving from one place to another. As time went by, society changed to an industrial society. Fewer people did physical labours as part of their work. Technology started being used, and physical labour was reduced. Jobs involved sitting for hours. Most of the manual labour that was earlier needed was reduced or completely negated due to the invention of great technologies. Thus, it became important to introduce movement as part of a regime or an exercise routine.

Like I mentioned before, the body needs to move. Movement may already be part of your lifestyle if you lead an active life; if not, you might have to introduce it in the form of exercise. Movement also has a strong relation to improving concentration and memory, increasing energy and enabling better learning. Have you ever sat through a long meeting or lecture and after a while felt restless? Your mind switches off and you no longer understand what is going on. Well, this is not only because the lecturer or colleague in front of you is boring, but actually because you are tired of sitting and need to start moving. Your mind and body are tired of being in one place, you need to get up and go for a walk and shake it off. After doing that, you can possibly go back and comprehend the proceedings of the day again. It almost feels like your brain is clogged and you can't hear, see or breathe properly any more. This alone tells us how important movement is to us.

To be more specific, movement is extremely important for the following reasons:

❖ **Maintains Body Weight:** Movement helps burn calories, which is essential for maintaining your body weight. To maintain your body weight, you must be able to balance the number of calories you take in (or eat) and the number of calories you burn. Movement and exercise in the form of weight training, Pilates, or any form of resistance training, increases lean body mass, which increases the basal metabolic rate, which, in turn, increases the number of calories burned.

❖ **Ease of Physical Movement:** We all know the saying 'Use it or lose it'. That is the case with movement too. If we don't move all planes, work every joint and muscle, soon, their functionality will reduce. It will be more difficult to move, you will feel weaker, movement will feel heavier and, soon, pain might also accompany every movement. Hence, keeping the body constantly moving is a necessity.

❖ **Improved Sleep:** Movement has been proven to improve the quality and quantity of sleep. It makes falling asleep easier. Active individuals tend to enjoy a sounder sleep and have less problem falling asleep than inactive individuals. Movement also helps reduce anxiety and hence promotes better sleep.

❖ **Internal Function:** The amount you move also affects your muscle development, hormones and cardiovascular functions. It improves blood circulation to all parts of the body and the body's ability to use oxygen. It slows the rate of decline in lung function.

❖ **Energy, Improved Mood and Stress Reduction:** When you do any type of physical activity and exercise in whatever form, you feel more energized, positive and less stressed. The body releases endorphins, which create a natural feel-good factor. However stressed you are, a good workout or a nice run will always make you feel refreshed and relaxed, and you will be able to face the challenge ahead of you. As you focus on movement and activity, the stressful things in life occupy your mind less and it becomes more focused towards the body. Movement has been proven to reduce depression and improve self-esteem.

❖ **Energy Levels:** The energy you have on a daily basis is directly related to the amount you move. The more active your lifestyle, the more energy you will have for daily activities. As I have mentioned earlier, the lazier you are, the lazier you will get. Many individuals have reported an increase in their energy levels after starting a fitness regime. They also feel more focused, happier and less fatigued.

❖ **Maintains Bone Density:** Movement is extremely important to maintain bone density. Weight-bearing movement especially helps in the stimulation of bone formation and hence can improve bone density. Movement can help prevent osteoporosis in women in the long run. Exercising helps to maintain, if not increase, bone density.

These are just some of the reasons why movement, especially weight-bearing movement, is extremely important. Movement at any age is essential. Staying active and keeping yourself moving should be as important as eating or sleeping. It is something you must do every day, in some form or the other.

There are various types of movement:
❖ **Lateral Movement** is associated with bending and moving from side to side.

❖ **Circumduction** is the circular movement of a joint, like the shoulders.

❖ **Flexion and Extension** refer to increasing or decreasing the angle of a joint. *Flexion* is bending or bringing the bones together. For example, the elbow is flexed when the hand is moved towards the shoulder. *Extension* is straightening or moving the bones apart. For example, the elbow joint extends to move the hand away from the shoulder.

❖ **Abduction and Adduction** refer to moving a body part towards or away from the midline. *Abduction* is movement away from the axis of the trunk, while *adduction* is movement towards the axis of the trunk. Lifting the arms to the side is a form of abduction, and bringing the arms back towards the midline is adduction.

❖ **Shaking Movements** are movements performed by an individual that shake the body or a specific part of the body. Shaking helps decrease stagnation in an area.

❖ **Passive Movement** is movement without any additional load or weight added to the body.

❖ **Resistance Movement** refers to the use of external force (like carrying a package or lifting weights) to increase muscular strength and bone density.

❖ **Aerobic Movement** refers to movement that increases the heart rate and the oxygen demand and intake, thereby conditioning the cardiovascular system. Aerobic movement can be accomplished with various activities including walking, running, biking, swimming, working the elliptical trainer, jumping, etc.

Your daily activity should have you move your body on all planes: sagittal, frontal and transverse. Human movement is divided into these three planes that help describe the movement. The *sagittal plane* divides the body into right and left. The *frontal plane* lies vertically and divides the body into the front and back, which are the anterior and posterior parts of the body. The *transverse plane* lies horizontally and divides the body into two parts—one above the trunk and the other below the trunk—dividing the body from the hip upwards and downwards. When you move a joint, it moves on all three planes of motion, but is dominated by one plane. For example, you would describe walking as a sagittal movement, while in reality, movement, is occurring on all three planes. It is important to understand movement and interpret it correctly.

Your daily activity and movement should involve stretching and releasing unnecessary tension in the body.

Studies have shown that, regardless of your age and prior physical activity, starting regular exercise can improve your health. Being active throughout your life is important, and it is never too late to start. Movement in any form from an early age is extremely important. Babies require some exercise to develop muscle and strength and also stay calm and get better sleep. The same applies to adults and the elderly too.

Exercising and movement during your teenage years and twenties are essential, as this age is usually when the lazy habits are formed. This is the age you start sitting around more than playing or running about. This is the age you study or work most of the time, limiting the time you spend outdoors or in playing games. This is the age where you must introduce working out as part of your regular routine. You should make it compulsory for yourself to work out. It should be a natural part of your day. Just as you cannot avoid going to college or working, you should not allow yourself to avoid working out. It is essential to keep moving at this age to form good habits, which will help in the long run.

I cannot emphasize enough how important stretching is. Let me put it this way. Let's assume someone is walking down a road in the rain, and the wet ground causes her/ him to slip. Now, imagine that the person who slipped has very tight muscles and not much flexibility. So when she/he slips—and especially if she/he slips and falls into a split—she/he will most definitely end up pulling a muscle due to lack of flexibility. Now, imagine that the same person knew how to stretch and was flexible—this would reduce the chance of injury. When the person falls, she/he will most likely be okay and move on. Simply put, what I am trying to say is that, first of all, stretching is important to help prevent injury. Several studies have found a significant relationship between stretching and the prevention of injury.

Stretching is as important as the exercise itself. It should be one of the first things you implement in your training programme. Mobility and flexibility work is so important that every sport has its own specific stretches. Stretching is probably one of the most neglected aspects of a fitness regime. Regular stretching is a must to increase flexibility and range of movements. Increasing flexibility through regular stretching will improve one's daily performance. Different tasks start becoming easier and muscles tend to have more endurance. An increased range of movement is the key to preventing injury and improving balance.

Stretching is also the key to releasing tightness in your body. It helps improve your posture, and an improved posture helps avoid unnecessary aches and pains. Stretching releases tight muscles and lengthens them so as to improve posture. A bad posture is usually the primary cause of unnecessary back pain and other aches and pains which can be reduced and avoided by stretching.

The soothing, calming effect of stretching helps relieve stress and helps you relax. When you stretch, you release the tight muscles that usually accompany stress and there is a lot of emphasis on breathing, which will help you relax further.

Types of Stretches

There are a few different types of stretching techniques. Here are the most common types of stretches, and the uses and benefits of each:

❖ **Static Stretching and Passive Stretching:** As the name suggests, *static stretching* involves holding a particular stretch in the same place for 20–30 seconds. Research has shown that holding a stretch longer than 30 seconds has no additional benefits. In a static stretch, you stretch your muscle to the furthest position, making sure not to overstretch. Feeling slight discomfort is okay, but the movement should not be painful. Once you reach this position, you must hold the stretch for 30 seconds. There is no bouncing involved. You should feel a mild pulling sensation, but no pain. This form of stretching should be done after a workout.

Passive stretching is holding a position with the help of some other part of your body, or of another person, or with the help of some external force. This is slow, relaxed stretching, and is very good to indulge in after a workout as it helps reduce muscle fatigue and soreness. For example, use your hands to hold a stretch in the same way that you stretch your hamstrings. Static and passive stretching are very similar and hence the term is often used interchangeably.

❖ **Active Stretching:** In this form of stretching, you stretch a muscle actively. This means that you hold a position with the help of the other opposing muscles. For example, in an active stretch, when you stretch your hamstrings and straighten your leg towards the ceiling, you hold it there with the help of your quadriceps. This means that, while you are stretching one muscle, you are strengthening the other. The theory behind this is that as one muscle contracts, the other muscle will stretch and relax. An active stretch is quite difficult to hold and is usually not held for more than 10–15 seconds.

❖ **Dynamic Stretching:** In a dynamic stretch, you are constantly moving. You move your body to gradually increase your range of movements and speed. A dynamic stretch does not involve going beyond your range of movements, but going up gently to the limit of your range. You must go to your maximum range and not push yourself to go beyond that. These stretches are usually performed before starting a workout routine or exercises and are sometimes used as a warm-up. An example of this sort of stretch is leg swings—where you gently swing your leg forward and backward—arm circles, or imitating a runner doing long leg-strides as warm-up and prep.

❖ **Ballistic Stretching:** This means forcing the body to stretch beyond its normal range of movements. This is usually done by bouncing—for example, bouncing your body to try and touch your toes. This form of stretching can cause injury. It is not considered the most ideal form of stretching. Only highly conditioned athletes should practise it.

❖ **Isometric Stretching:** This is one of the most effective methods to increase flexibility. An isometric stretch is when tension occurs in a muscle group without changing the length of the muscle. You can use a chair, a wall, a workout partner, or the floor to perform isometric stretches. These are needed as you can press into them or push against them to bring about a static contraction and an isometric stretch. For example, when you put your leg on a chair and stretch it by pressing into the chair, as if you wanted to bend your knee. Isometric stretches do not need to be held for more than 10–15 seconds and should not be done repeatedly on the same muscle group. Isometric stretching should be part of a cool-down rather than a warm-up.

❖ **Proprioceptive Neuromuscular Facilitation (PNF):** This type of stretching is the fastest and most effective way known to increase flexibility and range of movements. It uses a combination of passive stretching and isometric stretching. PNF stretching is usually done with the help of an exercise partner. It should be done slowly and carefully with the help of a trained professional. In this form of stretching, the muscle is first stretched passively, then isometrically contracted for a few seconds and then passively stretched again. This can be done a few times and then the muscle should be relaxed. For example, when someone helps you passively stretch your hamstring, you hold it there for a few seconds and then push into that person's hands for a few seconds, then you release and hold, and then, after 2–3 seconds, your workout partner will passively stretch you a little further.

These are some of the most varied but well-known techniques of stretching. You must consult your physician to find out which would be the most effective way of stretching for you. In general, though, if performed safely, cautiously and correctly, all the stretches can be useful in their own way. The bottom line is that if you want to stay pain- and injury-free, having a strong body is only part of that battle, and having a flexible body is also essential.

I am listing below some extremely relaxing, safe and easy-to-do-at home stretches:

❖ **Shell Stretch:** Sit back on your heels with your knees flexed (bent). Keep your legs slightly apart and flex your spine forward over your legs, keeping your arms relaxed in front of you or beside you. This stretch will help relax the muscles in the back. You must also relax your shoulders. This stretch will help lengthen spinal extensors.

❖ **Hip Release**: Lie down on your back, with your knees bent and feet hip-distance apart (the feet should be in line with the sit bones). Keep your spine in a neutral position and relax your arms by your sides, palms down. Inhale, release at your hip joint and drop one leg to fall gently out to the side, and then extend your knee, letting your foot slide away from your torso. Then exhale to medially rotate at the hip joint and pull the foot in towards the torso. Repeat 3–4 times on each side. Ensure that you do not tense the muscles in your hip joint, keep them relaxed, and let the movement flow. While doing one leg, ensure that the other leg does not fall to the side and that the pelvis does not rotate.

❖ **Spinal Rotation:** Lie down on one side with your knees and hips flexed, arms straight and forward at shoulder height, palms together. Keep your head relaxed. Inhale, reach your top arm towards the ceiling, and exhale, continuing to stretch the arm all the way up. Rotate the torso, let the chest open to the ceiling, and look up towards the ceiling. Inhale and then exhale to stay. Inhale once more and then exhale to rotate the torso back to the starting position. Keep your core engaged throughout the movement.

❖ **Cat Stretch:** In this stretch, you are on all fours. Keep your palms right under your shoulders, your knees flexed and under the hips. Keep your spine in a neutral position. Exhale to articulate your spine to flex it. Start with your tail bone, all the way to your head. Your spine should be completely rounded, but the shoulders should not have unnecessary tension. Inhale to stay and then exhale to release and go back to your starting position by articulating again from tail to head.

❖ **Roll Down:** Stand straight with your feet hip-distance apart. Ensure even weight on both legs. Starting with your head, roll down towards the floor, keeping equal weight on both your legs. Also ensure that the weight does not shift back to the heels—there should be weight on your toes too. Keep your hands relaxed. Roll down as low as you can go, inhale to stay there, and then exhale to roll up, head coming up last.

These stretches are extremely relaxing and, not only do they stretch different muscles, they also help in improving the mobility, flexibility and articulation of the spine. Like Joseph Pilates always said, 'You are only as old as your spine.' He also said, 'If your spine is inflexibly stiff at thirty, you are old; if it is completely flexible at sixty, you are young.' Having the ability to move freely throughout life is extremely important. You should be able to move your body in all the directions it is meant to move in—with control. You should be able to flex and extend the spine and you should also be able to laterally flex and rotate the spine. This can only be achieved by keeping the body moving throughout your life, not only regularly exercising it but also thoroughly and correctly stretching it.

My favourite regime that can give you all-round benefit is Pilates—for the simple reason that Pilates is injury-free and safe; it focuses on strengthening as well as stretching muscles, and emphasizes on improving posture and mobility.

It is something I believe everybody must try and do. Its comprehensive, all-round benefit has been proven to help many people around the world. A normal Pilates class comprises movement on all planes, with a focus on breathing, and yet it gives you a thorough full-body workout.

Now I am going to talk a little bit about warm-ups and cool-downs and their importance.

You exercise to lose weight, and to get fitter and stronger. Whatever be the reason to start exercising, you will not achieve anything sitting on a couch with a pulled hamstring, groin or some other muscle. These pulls are usually because people jump right into the exercise routine and avoid the warm-up period. A warm-up helps your body prepare itself for the exercise and thereby reduces the chance of injury. Not only does warming up help prevent injury, it also helps reduce aches and pains after a workout as it increases one's range of movements and reduces muscle tear. Warming up increases muscle temperature, which means that the muscles contract more forcefully and also relax more quickly. It reduces the risk of injuries, strains and pulls. Warming up helps lubricate the joints and helps improve your flexibility and range of movements. It also prepares your mind. It helps focus the mind on the routine ahead.

All the muscles that you are going to be using during the routine should be warmed up. Also, warming up the major muscles like your hips, calves, shoulders, chest and glutes, is important. There is no specific amount of time you need for a warm-up, but it usually ranges anywhere between 5–20 minutes, depending on the activity, sport or exercise regime.

A warm-up does not mean simply stretching and doing

static stretches before your workout. This could actually be harmful and cause tears and weird aches and pains. The muscle needs to be warmed up, not just relaxed. Hence, a dynamic routine is important in the form of a warm-up. You could do simple things like skip for a few minutes, or do some arm circles, leg swings and torso rotations.

Cooling down is also extremely important. It is one of the most neglected aspects of a session. A cool-down occurs immediately after your exercise routine and lasts for about 5–10 minutes. A good cool-down helps the body relax and slow down and also aids in faster recovery of the muscles. It consists of low-intensity movement and stretching. Stretching to help relax the muscles and increase flexibility is essential. Your cool-down must start immediately after you finish your workout. For example, if you have done a high-intensity workout and have been running, you can start your cool-down by reducing the pace to a jog and then a walk. Right after running you must be careful not to stop completely, sit down in your car and drive away. You have to give your body time to recover and relax. Slow down the movement and give your body time to understand that its regime for the day is over.

It is also important to stretch to release tension and relax the muscles. This is where you can do certain static stretches—for example, the simple hamstring stretch can be performed while sitting on a mat, legs straight in front of you, trying to touch your toes in this position. Ensure that you do not bounce as this is not the most ideal way to stretch. If you have a trainer or experienced person around you doing PNF stretching, it would be ideal if you were to enlist their help. Relax and stretch each and every muscle in the body, especially all the muscles that you have worked during the workout that day. This will help your muscles recover faster. The stretches you do should help relax your mind and should involve calm and steady breathing.

All aspects of a training regime are important: from the warm-up to the exercise routine as well as the cool-down. No part of your regime should be neglected. Now that you know the importance of movement and stretching, you should want to get yourself moving right now. Not tomorrow, not later today, but *now*. Let's not wait—or rather waste—another day.

4

MOVEMENT: GETTING OFF
THE COUCH

Got a break? Got a few minutes? Utilize them the best way possible. Do a quick 4-minute workout. This will refresh your mind, energize you and will get you to burn some serious calories.

All you need is 4 minutes. You can even do this 5 times a day. Taking a 4-minute break between work and any other routine is not difficult. Any workout is better than no workout. And by doing these quick workouts you are at least doing better than the person sitting on the couch. I am sure you can find this much time! Maybe you can do it first thing in the morning, just before you eat your lunch, or during any other little break, and you can squeeze this exercise in just the way you take a loo break. These workouts will get your muscles activated and get you off the couch. They will get you moving, which is essential. I do understand that, sometimes, because of a very hectic schedule, it is possible to miss a workout, and one's routine can go for a toss. But by doing these workouts you are keeping mind and body active and hence getting back into your regular routine later will not be difficult. For example, I will be honest and say I did miss my workouts on a few days while writing this book as I was writing, taking classes, setting up our new centre as well as going for meetings. What I did was that for every 1000 words I wrote, I got up and did a quick short-burst workout. This helped me energize, made me feel good, I found it easier to write, and I did continue to burn calories, work my muscles and stay moving.

The main key to losing weight, of course, is to burn more calories than you eat. If you cut down on your high-calorie food intake like sweets, biscuits, ice creams and cakes, you would have cut down on some major calories. This, accompanied by the 4- or 7-minute workout will help you lose some weight as you will be naturally ingesting fewer calories and burning a few more than usual. Another great thing is that some of these exercises, such as skipping, are cardiovascular exercises. These will increase your heart rate and you will therefore burn more calories. If you manage to work out for more time and keep this heart rate up for 20–30 minutes, you will not only burn a lot of calories but also improve your metabolic rate.

Metabolic rate is the rate at which the body burns calories. It is the amount of energy a person uses *at rest*, i.e., when she/he is not working out in any way. The reason the body uses energy even while at rest is to perform all its internal, natural functions such as breathing and circulating blood. Therefore, doing even short, high-intensity exercises will help improve your metabolic rate. You can run up a flight of stairs—this will increase your heart rate. Of course, doing cardiovascular exercises for a longer time is more beneficial, but even short bursts are great. If you manage to squeeze in a good 20–30-minute cardio workout, your metabolic rate will stay high even 24 hours after the workout. Isn't that great? It is possible to burn calories even while you are resting.

It is also important to build muscle mass as muscle burns more calories than fat. Hence, any form of strength training is important as this will increase your muscle strength and improve muscle mass, leading to more calories being burned, thereby giving you a better metabolic rate. But what we also must remember is that engaging in merely strength training is not good enough, one must do some form of cardio that increases our heart rate and challenges us. Both these things go hand in hand and both are extremely important. Just doing a million crunches will not get you flat abs—you need to burn the calories too!

Another important aspect to remember is breathing. It is extremely essential to relax the mind and body, to practise breathing exercises and to meditate. This will help you calm down, feel more relaxed and will also reduce stress. The reduced stress levels can help improve the way the body functions and hence can help increase weight loss. Also, breathing well helps reduce stress and anxiety, which often leads to bad eating. It will help you avoid overeating or eating junk and desserts. Meditating and deep breathing even once or twice a day can be extremely beneficial to your mind and body.

Here are certain common exercises you could do in 4 minutes.

❖ **Jumping Jacks:** Also known as 'star jumps', jumping jacks are a great way to get the heart rate up and burn some calories. When you do a jumping jack, you start with your arms down by your side and feet set wide apart, parallel to each other. To begin, jump up so that your feet open up wide and out, while your hands lift up sideways to about shoulder height, then return to the starting position again, thus alternating between the two positions.

❖ **High Knees:** Stand straight with your legs parallel and hands at hip height in front of you. Start jumping by switching weight between the two legs, almost as if you were running in the same place, ensuring that as you jump, your knee touches your hand each time. Try staying on your toes throughout to ensure least impact as well as quick movement.

❖ **Squats:** Stand with your feet open slightly wider than hip-distance apart and pointing slightly outwards. The weight of your body should be towards your heels and on the balls of your feet. Your toes should be able to wiggle during the entire movement. Look straight ahead and not down towards the floor. Have your hands straight out, parallel to the floor and your spine in a neutral position. Now, inhale to lower your body by pushing your hips out towards the back, ensuring that your knees do not turn inwards; they should be over your feet through the entire exercise. Try and go low enough so that your hip joint is parallel to the floor. Then exhale, press into your heels, and keep the balls of your feet on the floor as well, to straighten your knees. Keep your glutes squeezed and ensure that your back is in a neutral alignment throughout, and that there is no unnecessary rounding or extension in your spine.

❖ **Lunges:** Make sure your upper body is straight, shoulders relaxed and spine in a neutral alignment. Pick a spot in front of you and look straight at it, so that you don't keep looking down while doing this exercise. Step forward with any one leg and lower your hips until both your knees are bent at about a 90-degree angle. Ensure that your knees are aligned with your ankle and not turning inwards or outwards. Your front knee should not go beyond your ankle, and the back knee should not touch the floor. Then push back through your front leg, with more weight on the heels, to go back to the starting position.

❖ **Tricep Dips:** Place your palms on the bed or some sturdy bench or chair, with your legs on the floor in front of you. Lower your body slowly towards the floor until your elbows are about 90 degrees and then press up. Ensure that your shoulders stay relaxed throughout. Keep your core engaged while breathing in on the way down and breathing out as you press up.

❖ **Push-ups:** There are 3 ways you can do a push-up, depending on your strength level. The easiest is putting your palms against the wall, a little lower than shoulder level. It is perfectly okay to begin like this. Walk away from the wall, keeping your body in a straight line from head to toe. Slowly lean your entire body towards the wall while inhaling, and then exhale to press into your palms to push your body back up.

The second way of doing a push-up is to kneel, placing your palms on the floor. Again, ensure you stay long in this position. Do not sink into your back and ensure that you keep your core engaged. Lower your body very slowly down towards the mat, bending at the elbows—make sure you do not leave your bottom up. Exhale and press into your hands to push up.

The third kind of push-up is the full push-up: knees off the floor and legs straight so they can be either adducted or abducted, hip-distance apart. Ensure that your body is in a long line from head to toe; there should be no pressure on your lower back. Inhale to lower your body down towards the mat and exhale to push it up. The slower you go, the harder it gets. Start slow and build it up.

❖ **Ab Prep:** Lie on a mat, keeping your back in a neutral position, following the natural curve of your spine. Do not sink into the mat. Keep your legs hip-distance apart and knees flexed. Place your hands behind your head, gently supporting your neck. Inhale while staying down. Exhale and slowly lift your upper body off the mat, as though you were squeezing a pencil under your chest. Inhale to lower your body back on to the mat. Pulses in the ab-prep position, this is where you stay up and only move very little to keep squeezing that pencil.

❖ **Crunches:** Lie down on your back, knees bent and feet hip-distance apart, hands behind your head. If you have the core strength, you can do these without someone standing on your feet or with your feet locked under something. Exhale to engage your core and crunch and come up all the way, touching your elbows to your knees and then slowly going back down into the mat. Ensure you do not use too much momentum, try articulating and using the core correctly. Do not fall into the mat, but slowly roll into it on your way down.

❖ **Obliques:** The starting position is the same as in the ab prep. Inhale to lift your upper thorax (chest) off the mat. Exhale to rotate your upper thorax to one side, keeping your shoulders open and thinking about touching your ribcage to the opposite knee, then inhale to the centre and exhale to the other side.

❖ **Wall Sit:** This is a simple exercise. All you have to do is find a wall, stand with your back and head against it. Slide down the wall until your feet and knees are at a 90-degree angle. All you have to do is maintain this position. It is as if you were sitting on a chair.

4-MINUTE WORKOUTS

I give below a few examples of how you can combine the above exercises and get a quick workout in 4 minutes. These are just a few examples, but you can make your own combinations and permutations too!

Workout Routine 1
1 minute: Jumping jacks

1 minute: High knees
1 minute: Crunches
1 minute: Wall sits

Workout Routine 2

1 minute: Skipping
1 minute: Squats
1 minute: Skipping
1 minute: Squats

Workout Routine 3

30 seconds: Push-ups
30 seconds: Crunches
Repeat for 4 minutes

Workout Routine 4

1 minute: Ab prep
1 minute: Obliques
1 minute: Crunches
1 minute: Plank

Workout Routine 5

1 minute: High knees
1 minute: Squats
1 minute: Lunges
1 minute: High knees

Workout Routine 6

1 minute: Jumping jacks
1 minute: Tricep dips

1 minute: Push–ups
1 minute: High knees

Cardio Workouts

Tabata Workout
Duration: 4–8 minutes

Workout 1
20 seconds: Running on the spot—maximum intensity
10 seconds: Rest
20 seconds: Running on the spot—maximum intensity
10 seconds: Rest

Keep repeating the above till the 4 minutes are up. This is a great cardio workout and was designed by Dr Izumi Tabata for Olympic athletes. If you still have time and feel like going for one more round, then rest for 2 minutes and then again do a 4-minute workout. This workout is extremely difficult as it was designed for Olympic athletes. Hence, you could start with taking a 20-second break between sets instead of 10 seconds, and then build up to a 10-second break.

Workout 2
20 seconds: Walking lunges (right leg leading)
20 seconds: Rest
20 seconds: Running on the spot
20 seconds: Rest
20 seconds: Walking lunges (left leg leading)
20 seconds: Rest
20 seconds: Running on the spot

Keep repeating the above till the 4 minutes are up.

These exercises are all examples of 4-minute workouts. Now if you have a little more time, just a few minutes more, you could do a pretty intense workout! I give below a few examples of workout routines. These workouts would take anywhere between 7–15 minutes. In just this short time you can strengthen muscles, burn some serious calories and get an amazing workout.

Quick but Intense Weight-based Workout Routines
Duration: 7–15 minutes

Choose a pair of dumb-bells (weights) with which you can reach fatigue (meaning, a sort of decline in the ability of the muscles to generate force) in 10–12 reps (meaning, a repetition of a set of exercises), and tempo, with a 2-second lifting phase and 4-second lowering phase.

4-day Workout Plan

Monday: Chest/Shoulders/Triceps
1 minute: Chest press (lying on a box) OR Push-ups—
    10 reps
1 minute: Front shoulder raise—10 reps
1 minute: Lateral shoulder raise—10 reps
1 minute: Shoulder raise (overhead)—10 reps
1 minute: Triceps extension—10 reps
1 minute: Tricep dips—10 reps
1 minute: Abdominal crunches—20 reps
Total workout time: 7 minutes (approx.)

Tuesday: Legs/Back/Biceps

1 minute: Squats (with dumb-bells in hands) with feet parallel to each other—10 reps

1 minute: Squats (with dumb-bells in hands) with feet at 45 degrees (working the inner thighs)—10 reps

1 minute: Bent over rows (single hand)—10 reps

1 minute: Bent over rows (single hand)—10 reps

1 minute: Bicep curl—10 reps

1 minute: Hammer curl—10 reps

1 minute: Abdominal crunches—20 reps

Total workout time: 7 minutes (approx.)

Wednesday: Holiday

Thursday: Same set of exercises as Monday

Friday: Same set of exercises as Tuesday

FUNCTIONAL WORKOUTS

Workout 1

30 seconds: Jumping jacks

30 seconds: Push-ups

30 seconds: Squats

30 seconds: Abdominal crunches

1 minute: Wall sit

30 seconds: Abdominal crunches

30 seconds: Push-ups

30 seconds: Jumping jacks

30 seconds: Squats

30 seconds: Running

30 seconds: Abdominal crunches (with oblique twists; one side)

30 seconds: Abdominal crunches (with oblique twists; other side)

30 seconds: Jumping jacks

1 minute: Wall sit

1 minute: Plank

Total workout time: 9 minutes (approx.)

Workout 2

20 seconds: Medicine-ball squat with overhead lift (you may use a dumb-bell)

30 seconds: Abdominal crunches

30 seconds: Diagonal reach with dumb-bell (both sides alternately)

30 seconds: Leg lifts

30 seconds: Bicycles (lying on the back)

30 seconds: Squats

30 seconds: Sumo squats (with weights—optional)

30 seconds: Calf raises

1 minute: Arm circles (30 seconds right/30 seconds left)

30 seconds: Push-ups (knees on the floor)

30 seconds: Jumping jacks

1 minute: Plank

2 minutes: Wall sit

Total workout time: 10 minutes (approx.)

You do not burn enough calories, but it is better than doing nothing. And you will get stronger and feel more active, which is an added benefit. Doing these exercises should motivate you to do even more. It's about taking one step at a time. As you get stronger and these workouts get easier, you will feel like doing more, working harder and achieving more goals and targets. Once you see that the workouts are getting you more energized than tired and that they are making your mind more active, making you feel more positive, I am sure you will want to take yourself to the next level.

5

FUN: ACTIVITIES THAT BURN CALORIES

Fun activities that burn calories? That doesn't sound possible, does it? Actually, it *is* very much possible. Have fun when you work out, and it won't be difficult. Exercising doesn't necessarily mean you have to go to a gym, lift weights or run—there is a lot more that you can do. There are plenty of exercises that you can do at home, at least to begin with, and even outdoor activities. There are numerous activities that are fun, exciting, adventurous and most definitely not boring! All you need to do is find that one thing that interests you. Even simple things can burn a lot of calories. All you need to do is get up and get out. Sometimes it's hard to believe that some of the fun activities we are doing actually constitute a great workout.

Here are just a few things that you can try to get you started:

❖ **Shopping**: Let me start with the easiest activity for most girls—shopping! Oh, I think I can already see the smile on your face. Shopping in a mall or even roadside shopping can burn a lot of calories. When you are shopping, you are on your feet—walking around, standing and checking things out. You do not realize how time flies and walking for 3–4 hours non-stop feels like nothing. I know many girls who can start their day at 10 in the morning and can go on till 6 or 7 in the evening. Thus, this is an effective way to burn some calories and work the muscles in your legs. All you have to do is make sure the breaks you take in between do not mean eating a burger and fries or a pizza; instead, choose a salad or a healthy, tasty sandwich. This can easily be done once or twice a week. Check out a mall one Sunday and, on a weekday evening, check out the roadside stores—this way you will not get bored going to the same places again and again.

I have personally tried and tested shopping as a way of burning calories: it can burn up to 224 calories in one hour, which comes to 3.73 calories burned per minute. I decided to try this method on myself and went shopping to a popular mall in Mumbai with a few friends. We decided to check out some shoe shops, and try on some dresses and tops. Yes, we did end up buying a few clothes and shoes, but that is part of the fun, isn't it? Once we had the shopping bags, I decided to do some bicep curls and some triceps. So not only did I get a good leg workout and burn calories, but I worked my arms too. Yes, I did look a bit crazy, but so what? It was all part of the fun and ended up being a great workout too. Shopping is a pretty good workout to do every once in a while. And it's a great incentive to get yourself moving.

❖ **Skipping:** Skipping is easy and fun and can be done at home. It is the simplest thing to start with. All you need is a skipping rope and a little open space. The best surface to skip on would be a carpet or a wooden floor, or in the outdoors on mud or grass. Always wear sneakers or trainers while skipping. Another thing to keep in mind is the length of the skipping rope. If you stand right in the middle of the rope by stepping on it and holding up the handles, it should reach just below your shoulders. You can shorten your rope by tying a knot in it.

In order to skip correctly, make sure you hold the skipping rope handles in your palms, elbows tucked into your sides, and turn the rope smoothly with your wrists. Ensure that you do not lean forward or backwards and avoid landing heavy. Don't forget to breathe smoothly while skipping and also to keep your core engaged and back straight.

You can do these different types of skips:

• **Normal skips:** These are regular skips on both your feet, jumping smoothly and steadily. Keep your back and head straight while jumping. Land soft on your toes.

• **Side to side:** Do the same thing as in normal skipping, but jump a little to the left and then to the right. This helps activate and work the abductors and adductors.

- **Forward and backwards:** Jumping forwards and backwards will help activate your glutes and hamstrings more.

- **Running:** Shift your weight from one foot to the other while skipping; this will give you a sensation of running.

- **High knees:** As the name suggests, skip while lifting your knees high. Every time you jump, ensure you lift your knees up.

- **Butt kicks:** Try skipping while lifting both your legs up to kick your butt. This is challenging as you will have to jump higher and land quicker.

- **One foot:** Jumping on one foot is extremely challenging. It works the leg unilaterally and tones it. Jump on any one foot for at least 50 skips.

- **One foot front and back:** Same as the double leg forward and back; jumping on one leg will only make it a little tougher.

- **One foot side to side:** The same as the side-to-side double-leg skips.

- **Double unders:** Try passing the rope under your feet twice each time you jump.

- **Rope backwards:** Want to challenge your coordination skills a bit more? Try circling the rope the other way. Be careful not to trip.

- **Circles:** Jump in a circle clockwise and then anticlockwise to work the glutes, abductors, adductors, quadriceps and hamstrings simultaneously.

In just 10 minutes of skipping, which included a 20-second break every 2 minutes, doing the regular skips, front and back, side to side and single-leg skips, I burned 101 calories. That is 10 calories a minute, which is excellent!

❖ **Cycling:** This is something I love doing. If you have some open space like a park, a promenade or a building compound, I suggest getting out and cycling. Make sure you get yourself a good bicycle and are prepared to sweat a bit. Wear protective gear while cycling. Wearing a helmet is a must, of course, and it is advisable to wear knee pads and elbow pads too. Cycling can be done any time, as long as you are not cycling on a busy road. If you manage to rise early and cycle—trust me on this—your day will be brilliant. Watching the sunrise as you cycle, and feeling the early morning breeze and peace, especially in the city, is a sheer delight. I love going cycling from 6–7 in the mornings, and I usually cycle on the road next to the promenade. I cycle on the Bandstand and Carter Road stretch in Mumbai, early in the mornings. With the fantastic view of the sea coupled with the fact that this is the only time you can actually hear the waves and truly feel the breeze, you feel like you're in heaven, at least for a while.

You can go cycling alone or with friends. Make a cycling group so that you can try new routes and go farther. You can also join an existing group and make new friends along the way. Meeting more cyclists will motivate you to go out more, and working out will start becoming a fun activity. Cycling has many benefits, one of them being, as already stated, that you can actually make some new friends. Other reasons to cycle include the obvious fat loss that comes with it and muscle strengthening and toning. You work the muscles in your legs, which include the calves, hamstrings, glutes and quadriceps; you also work your arms, core, and back muscles to steer your cycle and stay upright, while working the extensors in your back. Also, if you stand and peddle, you will engage your core and work the triceps. You can burn up to 462 calories in an hour of cycling. Another advantage of cycling is that if you are overweight or new to the fitness world or have joint issues, cycling is a low-stress activity and is therefore relatively safe to do as the saddle bears most of the weight and the stress on your joints is reduced. It also reduces the stress on your ankles, knees, hips and spine.

You can cycle to places instead of taking a car—you will thereby cause less pollution and will also probably get there faster, considering the traffic situation these days. Like any other exercise, cycling will give you a lot of energy and will also help you get through the day. A good way to burn more fat while cycling is doing interval training, which means you cycle fast and hard for a bit and then at a slow steady pace. This could be one minute of fast cycling, alternated with one minute of slow pedalling. The pace and intensity of your workout will depend on how often you can go cycling. If you are going just twice a week, then work hard and give it all you've got—I would say cycle like you've stolen something! If you have time to go more than 4 times a week, then you do not need to push yourself too hard; you can cycle at a medium pace and sometimes just leisurely, and enjoy the view. This is definitely a must-try activity.

❖ **Dance Classes:** Dancing is one of my other favourite activities. Dancing is so much fun, and there are so many different forms of dancing. This is another activity that will help you get out, move, meet new people and make new friends. Once the music is on, I just want to move and, depending on the music, jump! You activate your whole body while dancing, from the head to the toes, literally. Dancing helps build muscle, gets you a lean and toned body, and also improves your flexibility, stamina, balance and endurance. You will build lean muscles, which means you will burn calories even when you are not working out. Dancing will also improve coordination, and work your mind and body. The fun, relaxed element of dance gives you an uplifting feeling that helps reduce stress.

There are plenty of dance classes around, and there are many different forms you can learn. You can join traditional Indian dance classes teaching Bharatanatyam, Kathak, Kathakali, Kuchipudi, Odissi and Mohiniyattam. I love watching Indian classical dances, and I find it extremely challenging. It is definitely something I would want to pick up someday. It is simply beautiful and, being Indian, I think we should all appreciate the classical dance forms and try learning them when we can.

Some Western dance forms that you could try are:

- **Freestyle:** As the name suggests, this dance form enables you to move freely and in the full range of motion. This is usually practised with loud, fast–paced music, thus making you shed calories and, at the same time, toning your muscles.

- **Tap:** This involves quick movement, especially of the feet. This form of dance tones the legs rapidly and gives great shape to your calves and thighs.

- **Jazz:** It can be fast, challenging and crazy, but the lovely music in a jazz class is what makes me love it the most. It really works your legs and core. I did a low–to–medium–intensity jazz dance class before my performance and found that I had lost 780 calories in 90 minutes—which means I burned 8.67 calories per minute, which is approximately 520 calories an hour, and 962 calories in 130 minutes. Post the dance class I was still burning 4.55 calories a minute even 40 minutes later. My average heart-rate while dancing was 134.

- **Contemporary:** Not only is this one of my favourite dance forms but it is also an extremely effective workout. This dance form is great for toning each and every muscle in the body as well as shedding a lot of fat. It involves twists, turns and all sorts of movements. You have to do floor work as well as jumps and quick movements. Your weight is on your arms a lot of the time, giving your arms a great workout, and the movement also involves breathing and keeping your core engaged.

- **Ballet:** This dance form is technical and beautiful. It tones the legs, works the arms, and improves posture and confidence. It is a great workout indeed and, once mastered, it is one of the loveliest dance forms.

- **Belly Dancing:** Oh, this is so much fun! Challenging and quick, this form of dance involves a lot of waist and hip movement. You will definitely tone your core, strengthen your lower back and increase the range of movements around the lumbopelvic region. It burns a good number of calories and is a marvellous way of working out and enjoying yourself at the same time. This too is something I have tried and thoroughly enjoyed. I have even performed this on stage. It challenged me and gave me a lot more confidence in my dancing abilities.

- **Hip Hop:** This involves quick movements. It works your abs, legs and even the arms. It gives you that fun feeling and makes you feel like a star. I love it and find it exciting. Sometimes, the movements can be quick; other times, they are slow and controlled.

- **Salsa:** Move it! That's what salsa is all about. It's sharp, it's sexy, it's superb. It involves a lot of waist movement, lifts and spins. It is quick and fun, it burns a lot of calories.

- **Jive:** It has a lovely bounce and groove to it. It involves sharp movements, and spins and twists, working the arms and legs. Dancing with your partner is also a lot of fun. Sometimes you get to dance with many different people, which is a great way to improve your dancing skills and also helps adjust to different people's techniques.

- **Bollywood:** Burn some major calories with this dance form. I think this is a lovely mixture of everything. Do some *latka*s and *jhatka*s, sometimes slow, other times fast. Sometimes you dance with someone and other times alone. But this form of dance definitely keeps you moving. The pumping music usually played in a Bollywood class is a lot of fun and even if you have not learned the steps yet, you already want to start moving.

Try all the dance forms or master one. Either way, dancing is simply superb!

- ❖ **Hula Hoop:** Get out the inner child in you! Remember how much fun the hula hoop used to be? Well, no surprise, it still is a lot of fun and a great way to shed some weight. You can hula-hoop any time, anywhere and anyhow. Hula-hooping is a growing trend worldwide. Many celebrities credit their bodies to hula-hoop exercises. You can get a full-body workout just using it. Starting with the core and using the rectus abdominis, transverse abdominis and obliques, and also using the quadriceps, glutes and hamstrings, you can work and tone the muscles in your arms. The hula hoop can be effectively used for a full-body workout. Hula-hooping is an effective way to tone up.

There are different methods you can use and several exercises you can do with the hula hoop to concentrate on different parts of the body. Here I list the different exercises that you can do using it. You can always mix them up to get a full-body workout. Don't forget to put on some fun music!

- **Side to Side:** This is the classic, basic move. Hold the hoop at waist level. Start by using your hands to set the hoop in motion by rotating it one way. Now, to keep the hoop in motion, keep moving your waist from side to side. You can do this for one minute, take a 10-second break, and then start again by trying to push the hoop the other way. Do it for one minute and then take a 10-second break. Or simply do it for 2 minutes one way and then take a 20-second break.

- **Front and Back:** Stand with your right leg in front and left leg back, not too wide apart. Start by using your hands to set the hula hoop in motion. Move your body front and back to keep it going. Do this for one minute, and take a 20-second break with the right leg in front. Then do another minute with a 20-second break with the left leg in front.

- **Ninja Passing:** Stand with your legs hip-distance apart. Hold the hoop in one hand. Twisting your torso, pass the hoop to the other hand. As your torso rotates, you pass the hoop from one hand to the other. Do this for one minute and then take a 20-second break.

- **Squats with the Hoop:** This is a little challenging, but a lot of fun. Stand with your feet a little wider than hip-distance apart. As you hula-hoop, move your waist from side to side and do squats. This requires coordination and control. The motion should be as if you were sitting on a chair. Do it for one minute and take a 20-second break.

- **Basic Passing:** This involves rotating the torso completely and passing the hula hoop from behind your back from one hand to the other. Do 2 sets to ensure you pass the hoop both ways—one minute and a 20-second break from the right, and one minute and a twenty-second break from the left.

- **Lunges with the Hoop:** Lunge forward with one leg, keep the hoop in one arm and do arm circles. If you are lunging with your right leg, keep the hoop in your right arm. This way, you work your legs and arms simultaneously. Do one minute with the right leg in front and the hoop in the right arm, then take a 20-second break, and one minute with the left leg in front and the hoop in the left arm, then take a 20-second break.

- **Side to Side:** This is the same as the first exercise. Do 2 minutes and then take a 20-second break.

- **Basic Passing with Lunges:** The basic passing is the same as the fifth exercise; the only difference is that this has to be done with lunges. Do lunges for one minute with your left leg in front and right leg at the back, then take a 10-second break; then your right leg in front and left leg at the back for one minute and a 10-second break at the end.

1) Back stretch with hoop: Do this for 10 seconds.

2) Side stretch: Do this for 10 seconds.

Total workout time: This consumes 18 minutes only! While doing this, I burned 105 calories, which clocks in a rate of approximately 6 calories burned a minute. My average heart-rate was 115. I did the workout at a moderately easy pace. This workout can be repeated thrice to make it a complete one-hour workout and can also be done at a faster pace so that you burn more calories.

❖ **Dog Walking:** Walking your dog—if you have one, of course—is a fun way to get out of your house and take a good walk. A dog is your best companion. You can go out at a time convenient to you, and man's best friend will be ever ready to keep you company. Not only is this a good way to keep moving in the day, but seeing that adorable, happy face will give you a different high. Their wagging tail, as you get them ready to go, and their happy barks are the added perks when you take these delightful creatures outside. The other fun thing is to watch the cute, little things they do along the way. They are inquisitive by nature, and seeing them explore the surroundings is another treat. If you have a healthy, fit dog, you can even go for a jog with your pet. You as well as your dog need exercise, so not only will you benefit yourself but you will also be helping your best pal stay fit. Just a warning though—different breeds of dogs need different amounts of exercise, so please do not overwork your furry friend.

❖ **Swimming:** The beauty of swimming is that it burns fat, helps you lose inches, and gets you stronger and toned—all this, without putting any impact on your joints. Swimming is something you can do at any age and throughout your life. If you don't know how to swim, it's never too late to start. Swimming is relaxing and fun and yet helps you burn some serious calories. Water neutralizes gravity, because of which you feel weightless in water, making the otherwise-strenuous activity easy on your joints. But water is denser than air, so swimming is like resistance training—you have to work hard to stay up and to move forward, which is how you will work your core, glutes, shoulders, arms and back muscles.

The four main swimming strokes are freestyle, breaststroke, backstroke and butterfly. In all the strokes, you work your arms, legs, core and back. In freestyle and backstroke the obliques are used more as they help with the rotation of the torso. The hip flexors are constantly working to help maintain a steady and powerful kick. In the butterfly stroke, there is a lot of emphasis on the lower-back muscles and also on the glutes. The breaststroke works the chest muscles, glutes and the quadriceps when doing the frog kick.

Try going for a swim at least thrice a week. Remember to warm up your entire body before you swim as the large range of movements during swimming means you need your muscles to be warm, long and flexible. Start your swim with a few relaxed lengths and then push yourself to go faster. If you are a beginner, start with doing a few lengths and take a short break between them; as you progress and start swimming more often, try reducing the breaks and swimming non-stop. As you advance, you will find that interval training is a great way to burn fat. Do a few lengths at a fast pace, then one relaxed length, and repeat.

Other things you can do in the pool include aqua aerobics and aqua running. Aqua running is basically running in a swimming pool—it's deep-water running. There's no impact on your joints and it is a great way to tone your muscles and to get almost the same benefits as actual running. If you practise aqua running, the form in which you run should be the same movement imitated in the water.

❖ **Skating:** Many of us have gone skating at some point when we were young. Skating is a great way to get out, feel the heat and get moving. Roller skating is considered an aerobic fitness sport. It is a cardio activity that helps you burn fat and gain muscle. Roller skating is especially good as it is a low-stress form of exercise, so there is less stress on your joints. Skating helps build muscles in the lower body; these include your calves, glutes and thighs. It works your arms and core muscles as you have to balance your body as you move. Skating also improves your balance and coordination. There are many different types of skates, so make sure you get the right pair for yourself. When you skate, ensure that you wear comfortable, protective gear, such as elbow pads and knee pads. You can also wear a wrist guard and gloves. Wear a helmet to be on the safe side—as I always say, precaution is better than cure. When skating, stay as low as possible and keep your knees bent comfortably because this helps increase balance. Keep your arms by your side and slightly in front of you. Learn how to skate on a smooth surface, in an area with little or no traffic (human or vehicular). When you feel confident, you can move out a bit and be a little more adventurous. When I was young, I was a real nuisance, skating around my house and round and round the dining table, refusing to take my skates off. But that's where I learned how to skate and then got out and went skating in my neighbourhood. When I went with my friends, we would race and try and skate up and down a slope; even falling while skating was part of the fun.

❖ **Trampoline:** Jump the fat away. Trampolines are so much fun, have less impact on your joints, and are a great way to work out. Ensure you have enough space, really high ceilings, or an open area, which is even better. You don't want to hit your head on the ceiling and hurt yourself. Start slow. Do small jumps on the trampoline. Start with your legs a little apart and arms by your sides, and do small, relaxed jumps. You can even prance (meaning, a movement with high, springy steps; it is like moving in a joyful manner) on the trampoline. This means you are running in one place, alternating the weight between your legs. Keep your hands on your waist and your core engaged. Another exercise you can do is a jump that turns into a squat. Jump up and land with your feet about shoulder-distance apart and in a squat position; you can do this 20 times.

❖ **Horse Riding:** I keep repeating this, but horse riding is one of my favourite activities. I have always said that having a workout buddy is fun, supporting and motivating. And who can be a better workout buddy than a horse! I know it is not as easily accessible as the other activities, but if you can join a local horse-riding club, ride your own horse (if you are fortunate to have one), or ride a friend's horse, then there's nothing as wonderful as horse riding. It works the mind and the body, the muscles of your arms, legs, inner thighs, quadriceps, and your core and back muscles. It helps build coordination and balance. It will also improve your concentration and posture, give you energy, and make you feel relaxed after your ride. Horse riding requires strength and endurance of all types of postural muscles. You must stay alert and aware. Riding involves sitting in a static position during a leisure ride or dressage (which means sitting straight with a good posture for an hour, allowing only subtle movements in the body). This may seem easy, but sitting with a good posture for a long time actually involves working the postural muscles, and can be extremely difficult.

There are also dynamic movements while horse riding, like when you are jumping or playing polo. You can never get bored of horse riding; there is always something new to learn. Riding different horses helps you learn new things and can be quite a fun experience. I have ridden a few different horses, some of whom I will never forget. There was one horse who loved to lie down. I was sitting on him and he decided to sit down and chill; I must have been really boring! I had to learn how to keep him awake and moving. Then there was this other horse that always wanted to go into a canter (which means a sort of run before a gallop), and I had to use my arm strength and keep him tight and slow. It is interesting to see that different horses behave differently, which means one also behaves differently on different horses. There are many things you must and can learn about horse riding. You have to learn how to move and stop correctly, trot, canter and gallop. You can learn various games like pole bending, barrel racing, or riding a dollar. You can also engage in more serious horse-riding sports such as showjumping or polo. When I went horse riding for 30 minutes, I burned 286 calories, and my average heart-rate was 118. I was trotting as well as cantering that day.

❖ **Cleaning the House:** Yes, I *am* really listing housecleaning as a fun activity. For starters, it will burn more calories than sitting on the couch. You could even leave your favourite show on while cleaning—at least this will keep you moving. You could start with vacuuming the floor: the forward-and-backward movement can help you engage your core muscles and use your arms as well. Sweep the floor while squatting rather than while bending down as this will work your leg muscles as well. Make sure you use both your arms evenly. Cleaning the windows and dusting will work your arms. If you are washing dishes, do calf raises while washing. The key is making even small activities effective and fruitful. I renovated my hall and rearranged the furniture, and the calories I burned in that period totalled 156 calories, with my average heart-rate at 83.

❖ **Concerts and Parties:** Oh yeah, it's party time! Yes, I am telling you to go party. The first thing I should and must say is that you can party once in a while, but this does not mean drinking excessively and getting drunk or overeating junk food. Partying every once in a while is all right—you get out, you move and, if there is good music, you dance, all of which means burning some calories. Assuming you are not doing anything that is detrimental to your health, there is nothing wrong with partying once in a while. It's okay to go out with your friends, meet new people and shake a leg. I go out now and then, dance a lot and have a lot of fun, though I do not drink or smoke. Trust me, it's mind over matter. If you want to have fun without drinking or smoking, you will be able to do so. In one hour of partying, in which you dance moderately, you will burn approximately 342 calories. If you do go for a party, remember to have fun and dance. After a night of partying, it is very easy to want to have some unhealthy greasy food, but choose tasty, healthier options instead. Do not get caught up in peer pressure—be your own boss and do what is right for you. Follow these few simple directions and you are good to go!

❖ **Playing on the Wii or Xbox:** Surprised? But playing these games can actually help you lose weight. Some of these games get you up and moving, and actually let you have some real crazy fun. You can play alone and have a blast or call some friends over and have even more of a blast. I love playing on the Wii and we even have it at our studio; we often make clients play on it as a change. This helps them stay motivated, as it is an amazing change from what can otherwise be a regular, boring routine. Playing on the Wii can be quite a calorie-burner, and the excitement of it is a great stress-buster. Of course, to burn calories you must play games that require you to stand and move about. Play in competition mode and see how much you enjoy yourself while burning calories.

As you can see—and, hopefully, believe—it is possible to do fun activities and lose weight. All these activities are movement-oriented; some are subtle, while others are more rigorous, but all of them get you moving. You should try at least a few of them to keep things interesting, so that you never get bored. Just keep it going and keep exploring. Move it before you lose it!

When I did nothing for one hour and sat on the couch and watched television, I burned only 88 calories. Thus, doing any of the simple, fun activities I have mentioned above can make you burn a lot more calories, and you will find yourself enjoying these activities and also gaining strength.

6

STEALTH: SNEAKING EXERCISE INTO YOUR DAILY REGIME

You will find that in the hustle and bustle of today's world, the major problem faced by exercise enthusiasts is lack of time. The reason why many people stay away from the gym is because they feel that to achieve a good fitness level, they would need to spend at least 75–90 minutes in a gym, 6 times a week. This is entirely untrue. What you need to do is merely use the KISSS principle: Keep It Safe, Simple and Smart.

A relatively good level of fitness can be achieved by working out 3–4 days a week for about 45 minutes or so, i.e., 20 minutes of cardio and 20–25 minutes of strength training. This should be coupled with reasonable eating habits, i.e., a routine that usually avoids sweets and fried stuff and incorporates more salads, fruit, lentils, walnuts, curd and milk; you can refer to the next chapter, where I have discussed nutrition in some detail. The time spent working out 3 times a week would approximately amount to 40 minutes per workout multiplied by 3 days (per week), i.e., only 120 minutes or 2 hours per week.

Considering that humans normally sleep 9 hours (540 minutes) a day out of the 24 hours (1440 minutes) in a day, the time available for work, play, health and fitness is 1440 − 540 = 900 minutes per day. These 900 minutes multiplied by 7 (days of the week) equals 6300 minutes a week of waking time. All you need is to give yourself 120 minutes per week to spend on your personal health and fitness, which comprises only 2 per cent of your waking time. This is all that is needed in a week to achieve a reasonable level of fitness. Easy, right?

Yes, it might be easy to allot that much time per week. However, it is not that easy to decide how to go about your regime to get maximum benefits. You need to train smart, or else you will end up spending many hours at the gym, or within the four walls of your home and still be unable to achieve a fitness result anywhere close to what you desire.

Let's start by discussing a good 20–40-minute workout. As a precaution, it is always a good idea to speak to your doctor prior to starting any exercise routine and get his permission and/or approval, confirming that you are ready for the exercise routine that you have chosen.

It is advisable to wait for at least an hour and a half after eating a meal before getting into any sort of exercise programme. As a rule, the higher the number of calories ingested, the longer you should wait before you exercise.

A good way to start a fitness programme is by doing an easy home fitness-test as shown below:

TEST YOUR STRENGTH

	Excellent (seconds)	Good (seconds)	Fair (seconds)	Poor (seconds)
Wall sit	90	60	30	< 30
Abdominal hold	25	15	5	< 5
Push-ups (reps) (Modified for women)	25	15	5	< 5

Minimum Passing Scores

	Men	Women
Muscular strength		
- Pull-ups	3	30-second hang
- Squats	4 in 10 seconds	3 in 10 seconds
Flexibility		
- Toe touch (standing)	Fingertips on the floor	Palms on the floor
- Back raise (with hand)	+18 inches from chin to floor	+16 inches from chin to floor
Heart–lung efficiency		
Holding breath after running in place for 60 seconds	30 seconds	25 seconds

The above exercises in the tests are explained as below:

❖ **Wall Sit:** Sit against a wall as if sitting on a chair (with quadriceps parallel to the floor) and with back fully rested against the wall.

❖ **Abdominal Hold:** Stand on a mat, feet hip-distance apart, knees bent. Crunch up with eyes towards your knees, and stay there.

❖ **Pull-ups:** Hold a rod fixed above you and slowly pull yourself up, trying to get your chin to the rod.

❖ **Squats:** Stand with your feet slightly wider than hip-distance apart, feet pointing slightly outwards. The weight of your body should be towards your heels and on the balls of your feet. Your toes should be able to wiggle during the entire movement. Look straight ahead, not down at the ground. Hold your hands straight out, parallel to the floor, your spine in a neutral position. Now, inhale while lowering your body by pushing your hips out towards the back, ensuring that your knees do not turn inwards; they should be over your feet for the duration of the entire exercise. Try and go low enough, so that your hip joint is parallel to the floor. Then exhale, press into your heels, and keep the balls of your feet on the floor too, to straighten your knees. Keep your glutes squeezed and ensure that your back is in a neutral alignment throughout and that there is no unnecessary rounding or extension in your spine.

❖ **Back Raise:** Lie down on your stomach, with your hands beside your shoulders. Slowly press into your palms to extend your back.

Now that you have an approximate idea of where you stand, let's talk about what you can do to become fitter, stronger, faster and more flexible. I have explained the routines and the most common ways to train—this will increase your knowledge about fitness and make you more aware about what you can do. I believe it is important to know what you are doing and why you are doing it. Various kinds of exercise routines are available to the exercise enthusiast, some of which are listed below:

❖ **Cardiovascular or Aerobic Training:** You can do this on a treadmill, elliptical trainer or cycle, or by running outdoors, climbing stairs, in dance classes, or aerobic classes. You can play a sport like squash, tennis, badminton or football. Any exercise that raises your heart rate is called a cardiovascular exercise. The numerous benefits of a good cardio workout are:

  • *It is great for the heart.* Cardio makes your heart stronger, increases its pumping capacity and enables a stronger blood supply to the organs, so that they function to their full capacity. But this does not mean that you should begin with a dramatically strenuous cardiovascular workout programme because, in fact, this can potentially cause heart failure. Always begin with a slow-to-moderate pace for 20–30 minutes a day, 3–4 days a week.

  • *It results in weight loss.* Any form of cardio burns a lot of calories. The rate of calorie-burning is different for different activities, but it is well known that all forms of cardio burn calories.

- *It lowers the risk of obesity.* For instance, it reduces visceral fat, which lies in your abdominal cavity and surrounds the vital organs, causing Type 2 diabetes, high blood pressure, high cholesterol, and so on. Being physically active also reduces the risk of breast cancer and prostate cancer according to research done by several leading institutions.

- It elevates your mood, eases tension and promotes relaxation.

- It gives you confidence as it makes you look good.

- It reduces anxiety and depression.

❖ **Strength Training:** You can do this by using free weights at home; for instance, by lifting buckets of water or by using select machines at the gym. The numerous benefits of a good strength-training programme are:

- An increase in muscle size (if desired) and tone.

- An increase in lean muscle.

- Increased tendon, bone and ligament strength.

- Increased physical performance and appearance, leading to greater confidence in oneself; improved metabolic efficiency, i.e., more calories burned even while resting; and a markedly decreased risk of injury.

❖ **Functional Training:** The focus in functional training is on exercises that use multiple muscles and joints, at the same time improving your muscular endurance, overall strength, coordination, balance, posture and agility to get a challenging, effective and full-body workout as well as to prepare the body for everyday activities.

❖ **High-Intensity Training:** This seems to be the buzzword these days. It combines cardiovascular exercise and strength training. The idea is to have a workout that is *not* time-consuming, but is very time-efficient and effective.

WHAT IS CARDIOVASCULAR EXERCISE?

Any exercise that raises your heart rate is called cardiovascular exercise. The normal training zone for a good cardiovascular workout would be 60–80 per cent of your maximum heart-rate.

The best fat-burning zone (which is defined by weight loss) is said to occur when you train between 60–70 per cent of your maximum heart-rate. This has, however, changed over a period of time, and studies show that high-intensity cardiovascular training for weight loss is the best option, which means that there will be periods of 80 per cent-plus heart rate during exercise and 60 per cent heart-rate at rest. This stresses the cardiovascular system more than steady-state exercise.

Given below is the way to measure your exercise heart-rate:

$$\text{Heart rate at 60 per cent} = \frac{220 - \text{Age}}{60 \text{ per cent}}$$

So if your age is 20, then your exercise heart-rate would be:

$$(220-20) = \frac{200 \times 60}{100} = 120 \text{ BPM (beats per minute)}$$

$$\text{Heart rate at 80 per cent} = 220 - 20 = \frac{200 \times 80}{100} = 160 \text{ BPM}$$

You should try not to train at a higher heart-rate; for example, at 90 per cent of the maximum heart-rate for more than 30 seconds or so. However, training very briefly at a 90 per cent heart-rate is good for increasing your anaerobic capacity, which works well for a sprinter or marathon runner. But as a general rule, sticking to a maximum heart-rate of 80 per cent is safer and more beneficial.

How much time should you spend doing cardiovascular exercise? Studies say that you must spend at least 150 minutes per week doing moderate cardiovascular exercise (at 55–65 per cent heart-rate) or 75 minutes per week doing high-intensity interval training. The ACSM (American College of Sports Medicine) guidelines for cardiovascular training and cardiorespiratory exercise are as under:

❖ Adults should get at least 150 minutes of moderate-intensity exercise per week.

❖ Exercise recommendations can be met through 30–60 minutes of moderate-intensity exercise (5 days a week), or through 20–60 minutes of vigorous-intensity exercise (3 days a week).

❖ One continuous session and multiple shorter sessions (of at least 10 minutes each) are acceptable to get the desired amount of daily exercise.

❖ A gradual progression of exercise time, frequency and intensity is recommended for best adherence and minimal injury.

❖ People unable to meet with these minimums can still benefit from some activity.

General Guidelines for Choosing Intensity

In general, to achieve any appreciable benefit from cardiovascular exercise, you must work at an intensity of 60–90 per cent of maximum heart-rate. The intensities for various fitness levels are as under:

❖ Beginners: Train at 40–60 per cent of maximum heart-rate

❖ Average fitness levels: Train at 60–70 per cent of maximum heart-rate

❖ High fitness levels: Train at 75–85 per cent of maximum heart-rate

You should try to burn at least 300 calories per aerobic training session.

Types of Cardiovascular Training

There are many options available to you for doing cardiovascular training. Here are a few:

❖ **Low-intensity:** This sort of cardio training is good for beginners and is normally done between 40–60 per cent of maximum heart-rate. It is a continuous training method, lasting approximately 40 minutes, and can be done 3–4 times a week. It is a good way for beginners to start their way to fitness and is recommended for obese people and for those looking for fat loss.

❖ **Medium-intensity:** Once you are comfortable doing the above, it is a good idea to move up the intensity to a medium level, which would normally last between 30–40 minutes, at 60–70 per cent of the maximum heart-rate. This starts the slightly heavy-breathing phase and is good for fat loss and increasing your aerobic capacity.

❖ **High-intensity:** This training is normally done at approximately 85–90 per cent of maximum heart-rate and is also called the anaerobic threshold. At this stage, you will be able to hear your breathing, but you will not be gasping for air, and your heart-rate shoots up to 85–90 per cent of the maximum heart-rate—it is intense and demanding work. This sort of training is normally done from 5–20 minutes at a stretch, depending on your fitness level and the intensity of the workout. This sort of training should not be done until you are very comfortable with training at medium-intensity level.

❖ Some variations to the above training intensities are:

  • **Interval Training:** You can do aerobic interval training or anaerobic interval training.

    – *Aerobic Interval Training* means alternating between moderate- to high-intensity training; for example, walking for one minute and then running for 2 or 3 minutes, and then walking and running again, and so on. The timing of moderate- and high-intensity training can be adjusted to your fitness level. You can even do 10 minutes of running and 2 minutes of walking, and so on. You can do this programme for up to 20–30 minutes for optimum results.

— *Anaerobic Training* means training hard for short periods of time and then resting for the same amount of time or even longer. It is done at high-intensity, i.e., at 85–100 per cent of maximum heart-rate. This is a very demanding workout and *should not be done without supervision* and not for extended periods of time. The maximum you should train in this zone should be approximately 3–5 minutes. An example of training in this zone is a 30-second sprint followed by a 30-second walk and so on, for up to 3–5 minutes.

• **Fartlek Training:** This training means 'speed play' in Swedish. You play with the speed of your workout, and the resultant training is a combination of all the above. Here are a few examples:

— Try a 5-minute run followed by a 2-minute walk, followed by a 30-second sprint, followed by a 60-second walk, followed by a 6-minute run, followed by a 3-minute slow jog, and so on. Each session should last from 30–60 minutes, depending on your fitness level.

Interval Fartlek training: Here is a programme designed by my father and fitness expert, Samir Purohit:

Warm-up	5-minute walk, or slow jog at 5.5 kmph, at a 7 per cent incline
1.6 km	Run at 9.5 kmph at a 1 per cent incline
Rest set	Slow it down to 8 kmph and run for 3 minutes
Work set	Speed up to 11 kmph for 30 seconds
Rest set	Go back to 8 kmph for 3 minutes
Rest/work sets	Repeat the 3-minute and 30-second intervals until the clock reaches 25 minutes
1.6 km	Run at 9.5 kmph
Cool-down	Slowly jog for 5 minutes at 5.5 kmph at a 5–7 per cent incline.

The session will last for approximately 45–50 minutes.

Fartlek training can be a lot of fun as there is a surprise element in it due to there being no set routine.

❖ **Tabata Intervals:** This workout was designed to save time and also to give a great strength–and–cardio workout. The routine comprises high-intensity interval training and consists of 20-second high-intensity work followed by 10 seconds of rest. You need to do 8 such cycles. The time spent doing this routine would be 4 minutes, but believe me, these 4 minutes would be very taxing for your cardiovascular system.

The study done by Dr Tabata showed that this 20-second workout and 10-second rest routine gave a great aerobic and anaerobic workout, improving overall cardiovascular output.

Here are various aerobic activities that you can do using the above principles:

❖ **Walking:** This is probably the simplest of all aerobic exercises. It is a great way to start your journey to getting fit. A good idea is to start with, say, a 10–15-minute walk at a gentle pace and then increase the duration to up to 30–45 minutes. As you get comfortable with the duration, you can start increasing your speed of walking while reducing the duration to about 30 minutes. This can be done 3–5 times a week. The intensity of the workout can be low or high, depending on your fitness goals. It is important to use good footwear and to include a warm-up and a cool-down in your exercise routine.

❖ **Jogging or Running:** Incorporating about 20–30 minutes of this activity for about 3–4 times a week is good. You can begin by jogging and then increase the speed to a run. You can alternate between jogging and running, as mentioned in some of the principles above. It is important to use good footwear and include a warm-up and a cool-down in your exercise routine. This is important especially for your calves, lower back, quadriceps, hamstrings and hip flexors.

❖ **Cycling (indoors):** It is important to have good ventilation in the room. The height of the seat should be set such that your knees are slightly bent when you are peddling at 'max down' position.

❖ **Cycling (outdoors):** Here too you should observe some safety guidelines such as wearing a helmet and fixing a night illuminator on the bike and/or on your clothes.

❖ **Swimming, Rowing, Stair-Climbing and Step-ups:** These are other ways to work out. In swimming too, you can follow interval training. For example, do one lap at high speed and then do one relaxed lap. If you have no time—and even if you do—climbing stairs is a great way to work out. Use the staircase wherever and whenever possible. Run up a floor, then walk up a floor—and repeat. This is challenging and yet easily accessible and less time-consuming. You can also play sports like squash or football as they will increase your heart rate and give you a great workout, while still being a lot of fun. You will notice that when you play a sport, it is somewhat like interval training, as sometimes you need to go fast, while in between you can move slowly or take small breaks.

Now, we move on to strength training or resistance training. The ACSM guidelines for resistance training are as under:

❖ Adults should train each major muscle group 2 or 3 days each week, using a variety of exercises and equipment.

❖ Very light or light-intensity training is best for older persons or previously sedentary adults who are just starting to exercise.

❖ About 2–4 sets of each exercise will help adults improve their strength and power.

❖ For each exercise, 8–12 repetitions improve strength and power; 10–15 repetitions improve strength in middle-aged and older persons starting to exercise; and 15–20 repetitions improve muscular endurance.

❖ Adults should wait at least 48 hours between resistance-training sessions.

Strength training can have many routines; for example, one-set training (i.e., high-intensity training), 3-set training, multiple-set training, and so on. You can train all your body parts in one workout (i.e., circuit training), or train 2 or 3 body parts in one workout, or one body part per workout session, etc.

What is High-Intensity Strength Training?

❖ High-intensity strength training (HIT) reduces the workout time and increases the effectiveness and efficiency of a workout programme by maximizing muscle and strength gains.

❖ The fundamental principles of HIT are intensity, progression, duration and frequency. Exercises are performed with a high level of effort or intensity, where it is thought that it will stimulate the body to produce an increase in muscular strength and size.

Advocates of HIT, like Dr Wayne Westcott and Ellington Darden, believe that this method is more superior with regard to strength than most other methods which, for example, may stress lower weights with larger volume (i.e., repetitions and sets).

❖ Generally speaking, a HIT session will take you less than 30 minutes to complete. But these 30 minutes will be physically and mentally demanding in terms of muscle and mind effort.

❖ The basic concept of HIT is to extend the exercise set in some way at the point of muscle fatigue to achieve an even greater strength-building stimulus.

❖ Another equally productive procedure is to extend the exercise repetition by slowing down the movement speed.

Basic HIT Training Method

❖ *Number of repetitions:* 8–12 per set (You must reach fatigue at no more than 12 repetitions)

❖ *Number of exercises per body part:* 3–4 (If you do not have the time, even one set per body part is acceptable x 10–12 machines/exercises per workout)

❖ *Tempo:* 2 seconds in lifting (concentric phase)/4 seconds in lowering (eccentric phase)

❖ *Rest:* 60 seconds after each exercise. You can use this time to stretch the part just worked out in order to save time.

❖ *Total time for one round of circuit training:* 24 minutes

❖ *Number of days per week:* 2–3 or 3–4 days at the most.

❖ *Body parts trained:* You can train all the body parts each day (by circuit training), or the chest/shoulders/triceps on days 1 and 3, and legs/back/biceps on days 2 and 4, with abdominal and lower-back training on all days. In case you decide to train all body parts on a single day (through circuit training), then it is a good idea to train only 3 days a week because, due to the intensity of the training method, your mind as well as body will need a day's break to recover from this routine.

Let me give you a basic routine based on circuit training. The training can be done by doing just one round of all exercises or even 2 or 3 rounds of all the exercises as shown below. However, one round of the exercises mentioned below as per the principles mentioned above will help you achieve a reasonable level of fitness. Do remember that nutrition also plays a very important part in your achieving a reasonable level of fitness. These exercises can be done at home or at the gym.

❖ Leg extension (works the quadriceps)
❖ Leg curl (works the hamstrings)
❖ Leg press (works both the quadriceps and the hamstrings)
❖ Chest press (works the chest)
❖ Pec fly (works the chest)
❖ Overhead shoulder press (works the deltoids)
❖ Lat pulldown (works the upper back)
❖ Mid-row/compound row (works the mid-back)
❖ Tricep extension (works the triceps)

❖ Bicep curl (works the biceps)

❖ Abdominal (works the abdominals)

❖ Low back (works and strengthens the lower back)

This routine works all the body parts, is time-efficient (it takes less than 30 minutes, and in fact can be done in 24 minutes) and is an effective way to work out. It can be done at home or at the gym. Here are explanations of each exercise if you choose to do them at home:

❖ **Leg Extension:** This exercise can be done at home, sitting on a chair, putting weights on the ankles and lifting the lower leg parallel to the floor. This can be done using a single leg or both the legs at the same time.

❖ **Leg Curl:** For this exercise you should lie face down on a flat bench or bed, with weights around your ankles and then curl the ankles up by bending at the knee. Another way is to stand facing the wall, or holding a chair and curling one leg at a time by bending at the knee and trying to touch the back of your glutes.

❖ **Leg Press or Squats:** Start by standing and keeping your legs a little wider than shoulder width. Keep a chair behind you and then bend at the knees and just slightly sit on the chair (without completely sitting) and get up. Continue doing this for the repetitions decided above. Try not to allow your knees to reach too far ahead of your toes.

❖ **Chest Press/Push-ups:** Going in a part-plank (knees on the floor) or full-plank position, depending on your fitness level, bend at the elbows, move the chest towards the floor and rise.

❖ **Pec Fly:** Lie face up a narrow (shoulder-width) bench and stretch your hands (keeping your elbows soft) outwards and parallel to the floor. Bring the arms close to each other, right above the chest, and return.

❖ **Overhead Shoulder Press:** Standing up, hold weights (according to your strength), with your hands parallel to the floor and bent at the elbows. Lift the weights up towards the ceiling by bringing them close to each other and extending your hands fully (keeping the elbows slightly soft) and returning to the starting position.

❖ **Lat Pulldown:** This can be done by using a flex band— the types available are soft, medium, hard and very hard. The flex band can be tied to a doorknob or hook at about 6 feet. You should be positioned on your knees, with your hands fully extended upwards (keeping the elbows soft) towards the hook, with the flex band firmly in your palms. Pull the band towards your shoulder with your elbows opening outwards and parallel to the floor and return to the starting position.

❖ **Mid-Row/Compound Row:** This too can be done by using a flex band which can be tied to a doorknob. You should be seated on the floor with your hands fully extended (keeping the elbows soft) towards the knob, with the flex band firmly in your palms. Pull the band towards your lower chest with your elbows opening outwards and parallel to the floor (with palms prone, i.e., facing downwards) and return to the starting position.

❖ **Tricep Extension:** Position one dumb-bell overhead, with both hands holding the dumb-bell in a heart-shaped grip under the head of the top dumb-bell plate. Keep your elbows overhead, with the arms bent at the elbows towards the shoulders. Extend the arms fully upwards towards the ceiling and return to the starting position.

❖ **Bicep Curl:** Hold the bicep in one hand, keeping your hand fully extended towards the side of the hips. Then curl the dumb-bell by bending at the elbows and move the dumb-bell up towards the shoulder, keeping the elbow nicely tucked into the side of the body.

❖ **Abdominal:** Lie on the floor with your knees bent and hands behind your head (only for support). Contract your abdominal muscles by breathing out, and rise up from your head, keeping your lower ribcage grounded and crunched up.

❖ **Low Back:** Back extensions are probably the best. But take care not to extend your back too much. One safeguard would be to keep your pubic bone grounded while doing back extensions.

If you decide to train as per the 'push' and 'pull' training method, this entails push exercises on one day (such as chest followed by shoulders, followed by triceps), and then pull exercises (such as back and biceps) the next day. You can do leg exercises on this day even though they do not classify as pull exercises. You can train 4 days a week, for instance, training on Monday (push exercises), followed by Tuesday (pull exercises), then resting on Wednesday, repeating the same on Thursday and Friday, and resting again on Saturday and Sunday to get yourself ready for the exercise routine the following week.

It is important to know that in the push routine, when you exercise, you are training the chest, shoulders and triceps while doing chest exercises; you are training the shoulders and triceps while doing shoulder exercises; and then you are training only the triceps. This way, you fatigue the muscles more and there is better muscle activation and, hence, a better response to your training.

In the pull exercise routine, when you are exercising, you are training the back and biceps while doing back exercises and then only the biceps. Once again, this way, you will get better muscle activation and, hence, a better response to your training.

Here is a basic routine using the push-and-pull training method. You do this on day 1 (Monday) and day 4 (Thursday). Remember that day 3 (Wednesday) is a rest-and-recovery day.

❖ Push-ups
❖ Chest press
❖ Pec fly
❖ Front shoulder raise
❖ Lateral shoulder raise
❖ Overhead press
❖ Tricep extension (overhead)
❖ Tricep kick-back or tricep press-down
❖ Abdominal exercise: Perform crunches (till you are fatigued). While doing crunches, ensure that your pelvis

is stable and your feet are firmly grounded, with the knees bent while doing the crunches. Do not use your lower-back muscles to come up into a crunch.

❖ Low back (back-extension exercises): Do not come higher than your pubic bone, i.e., keep your pubic bone well grounded.

The approximate duration of the above routine is approximately 20 minutes. Not bad for an effective and efficient workout, right?

The exercises for day 2 (Tuesday) and day 5 (Friday) are as below. Day 6 (Saturday) and day 7 (Sunday) are rest days.

❖ Leg extension

❖ Leg curl

❖ Leg press

❖ Lat pulldown

❖ Mid-row/compound row

❖ Bicep curl

❖ Hammer curl

❖ Abdominal exercise: Perform crunches (till you are fatigued). Ensure that your pelvis is stable and your feet are firmly grounded, with the knees bent while doing crunches. Do not use your lower-back muscles to come up into a crunch.

❖ Low back (back-extension exercises): Do not come higher than your pubic bone, i.e., keep your pubic bone well grounded.

There are various HIT methods besides the basic routine shown above. Here, we try to extend the set a little longer to get more muscle activation. Note that the training principles will remain the same as explained before, i.e., with regard to the number of repetitions, sets and tempo.

- ❖ **Breakdown Training:** This involves taking a weight which will help you reach muscle fatigue in 10 or 12 repetitions—this is normally approximately 75 per cent of maximum one repetition, which is the weight that you carry for a maximum of one repetition. Now, lower the weight immediately by 10–20 per cent and try and lift the weights for, say, 2–4 reps, so that you experience muscle fatigue a second time, which would mean that you are recruiting more muscle fibre, hence enhancing muscle development.

  After 2 weeks of breakdown training, you should return to the standard (basic) training programme for 2–4 weeks, and then move ahead. This sort of training will be well received physiologically and psychologically, with further gains in muscle strength development, while reducing the risk of your being affected by the overtraining syndrome.

- ❖ **Assisted Training:** This is similar to breakdown training in theory, but there are two important differences:
  - You need a knowledgeable and cooperative partner/ trainer to give appropriate assistance when you reach muscle fatigue.

- A well-executed assisted-training set produces eccentric and concentric muscle fatigue.

In assisted training, you choose a weight with which you will reach muscle fatigue in 8–12 good repetitions, at the same tempo as explained before. The next step is to get manual assistance from your partner to lift a few more repetitions (2–4) after initial muscle fatigue.

A variation to assisted training is that your partner puts her/his weight on the weight stack and does not allow you to return the weights to the weight stack, i.e., you work on the lowering or eccentric phase.

After 6 weeks of assisted training, you should return to the standard (basic) training programme for 2–4 weeks, and then move ahead. This sort of training has the same benefits as breakdown training described above.

❖ **Pre-Exhaustion Training:** This is also called 'super sets', i.e., you train a body part up to a level of fatigue and then move to another exercise (with minimum delay), where you can train the same body part to a second muscle fatigue.

A good idea is to work a single joint muscle first (for example, the quadriceps) by doing 8–12 reps and then doing a multi-joint (compound) exercise to re-fatigue the muscle targeted by doing 4–5 good repetitions. The reason for this is that the fresh hamstring muscles assist the pre-fatigued quadriceps muscles, enabling you to perform a few high-effort leg presses that fatigue the quadriceps muscle fibres even more, enhancing the development of the quadriceps beyond standard training.

After 6 weeks of pre-exhaustion training, you should return to the standard (basic) training programme for 2–4 weeks and then move ahead.

Extending the Exercise Repetition: Slow Training

❖ Slow-movement speeds produce more muscle tension and greater muscle force.

❖ Slow training can be done by taking 4 seconds in the lifting phase and 6 seconds in the lowering phase.

❖ Super-slow training, developed by Ken Hutchins, is a strength-training technique that extends each exercise repetition to 14 seconds, i.e., 10 seconds in the lifting phase and 4 seconds in the lowering phase (slow positive emphasis), or 4 seconds in the lifting phase and 10 seconds in the lowering phase (slow negative emphasis).

❖ It is advisable to try and see that the set does not extend beyond 90 seconds because, if you went beyond it, you would enter the anaerobic phase and there could be a chance of injury.

❖ There could be between 4–6 repetitions per set.

Some important points to remember while doing slow training are:

• Have a trainer count out the seconds loudly to help you.

- Inhale and exhale as needed. You do not need to follow the normal breathing norms. Never hold your breath.
- Do 4–6 repetitions in case of super-slow training.
- Due to the reduced role of momentum, you will need to use less resistance for super-slow training as slower movement speeds produce more muscle tension and greater muscle force.

As the super-slow technique is physically and mentally demanding, performing 4–6 weeks' training periods alternating with 2–4 weeks of standard training is recommended. This reduces the risk of staleness and burnout.

Combined Strength-Training

This involves all the 5 high-intensity techniques because they offer a relatively low risk of injury and a relatively high rate of strength development.

You can also do a combined high-intensity strength training that involves all the 5 high-intensity techniques on a weekly basis, over a 6-week programme, i.e., you do the 5 workout programmes and follow them with a personal preference HIT workout.

The *expected* results over a six-week period (as mentioned by industry experts like Dr Wayne Westcott and Ellington Darden) are:

❖ An increase in weight load by 8–9 kg
❖ Add 1 kg lean (muscle) weight

❖ Lose 1.7 kg of fat weight, i.e., change of approximately 2.7–3.6 kg in body composition
❖ You are mentally fresh due to the continuous change in the exercise routine over the 6-week period.

There are many more methods of strength training:

❖ Multiple-set routines
❖ Training to muscle failure
❖ Tabata interval-training

Multiple-set Routine: This routine is probably the most followed in gyms and consists of a client doing 3–5 sets of various exercises.

This routine too can be done by working out all the body parts in a single day (3 days a week), or using the push-and-pull method of training (4 days a week), or doing a single body part a day (5–6 days a week).

As we are discussing ways to get moving, i.e., getting relatively fit, I would suggest doing only two of the options mentioned above—either working out all the body parts in a single day in a circuit form of training, or doing the push-and-pull method of training.

Circuit Training, 3-set Routine: You should start with a weight with which you can do 12–15 repetitions in the first set—this acts as a kind of warm-up for that body part. The second set should comprise approximately 10–12 repetitions, and the third should lead to muscle fatigue in approximately 8–10 repetitions.

If you have achieved a reasonable workout routine and wish to increase your workout intensity or workout time, you can start with some of these exercises:

You should rest for about 1 or 2 minutes between sets—you could use this time to stretch the working muscles.

- Leg extension
- Leg curl
- Leg press
- Incline leg press
- Calf raises
- Flat chest press
- Incline chest press
- Decline chest press: You should be careful about the weight you take, as too heavy a weight puts too much pressure on your shoulder joints, which could lead to shoulder problems.
- Pec fly
- Front shoulder raise
- Lateral shoulder raise
- Overhead shoulder press
- Tricep extension (overhead)
- Tricep dips
- Bicep curl
- Hammer curl

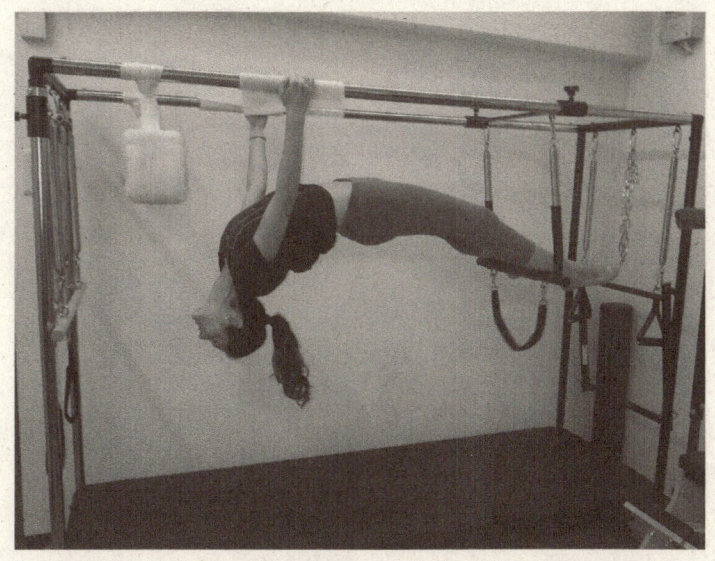

Bruna Abdullah practising the spread eagle to strengthen muscles after suffering from a slipped disk.

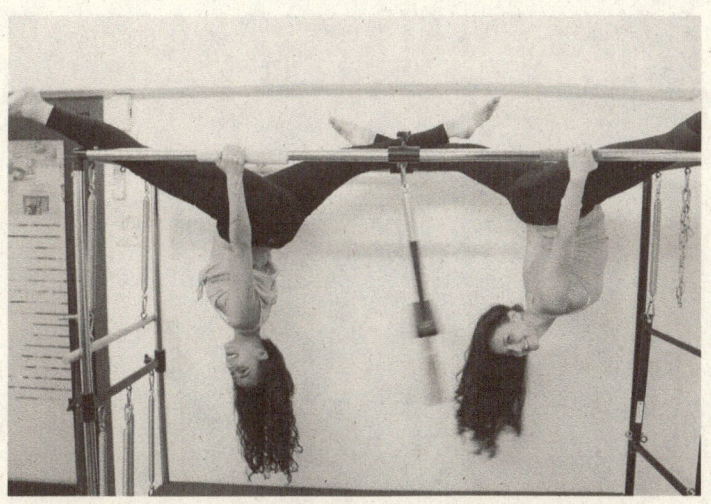

Elli Avram and Namrata doing the Pilates walkover on the Cadillac.

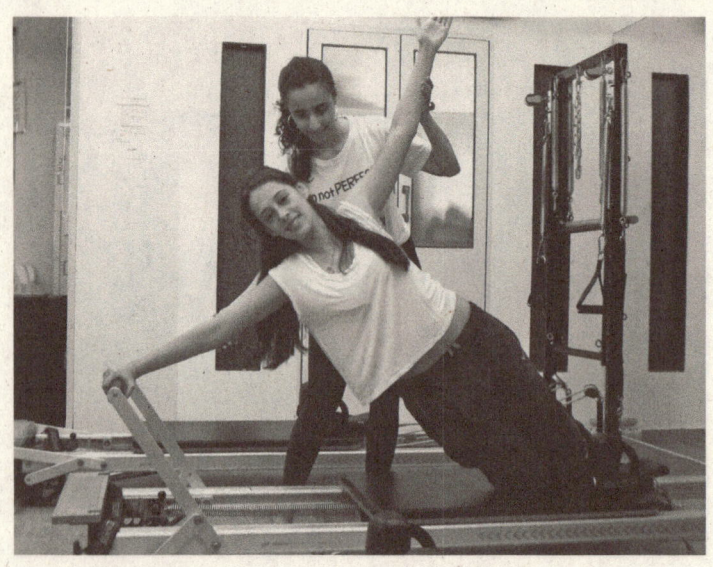

Hazel Keech doing the star prep on the Reformer.

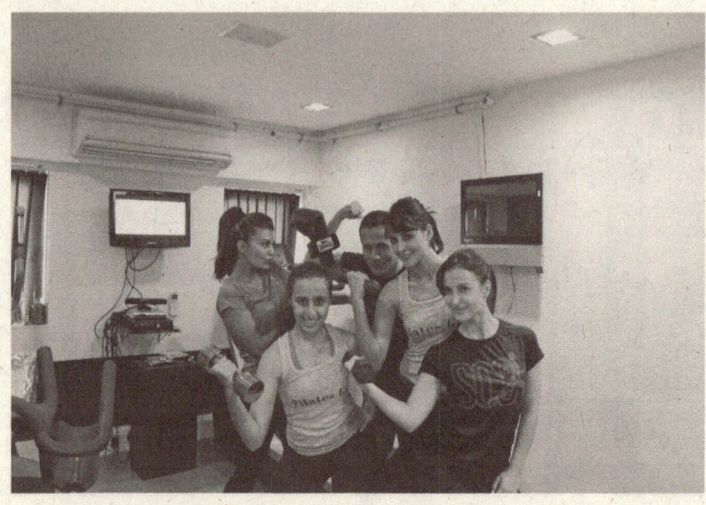

Jacqueline, Elli, Mandana and I with my father, Samir Purohit.
You must have fun when you work out!

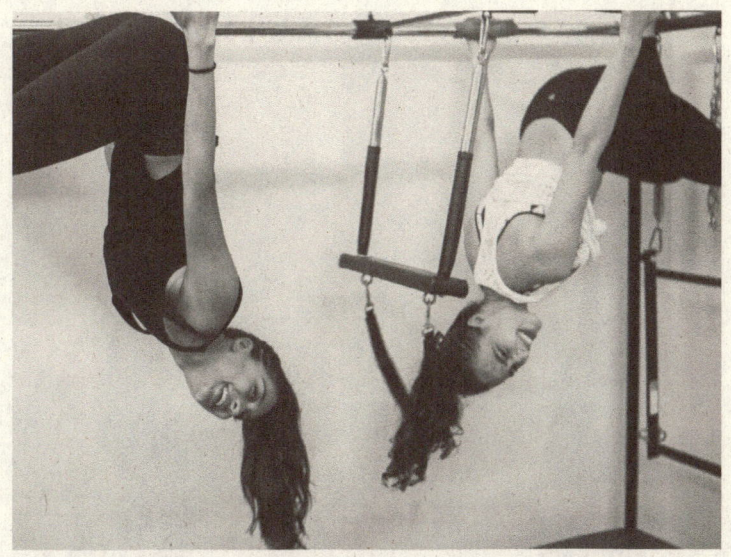
Monkeying around on the Cadillac: Lisa Haydon and Namrata.

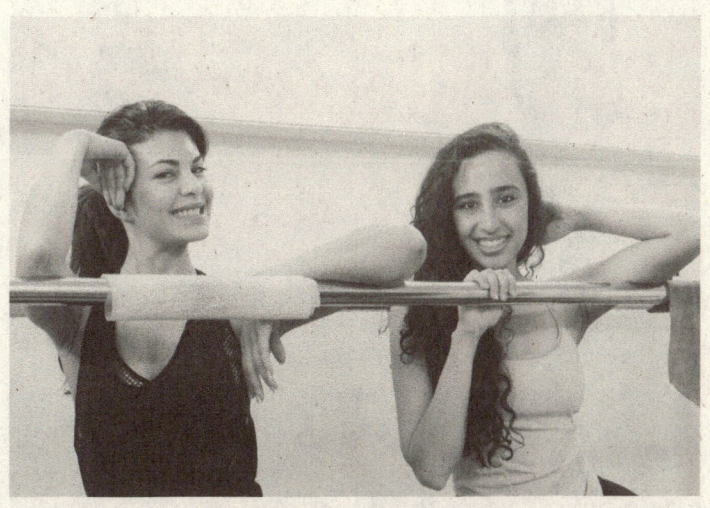
Namrata and Jacqueline.

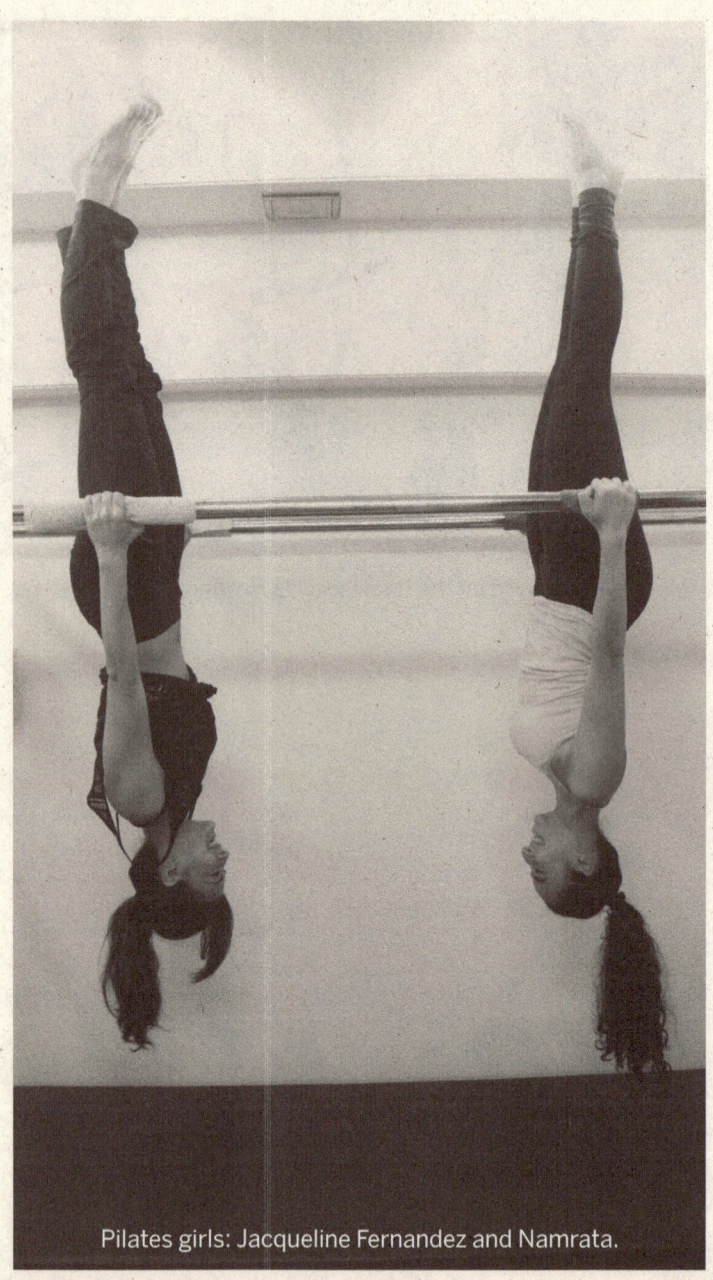

Pilates girls: Jacqueline Fernandez and Namrata.

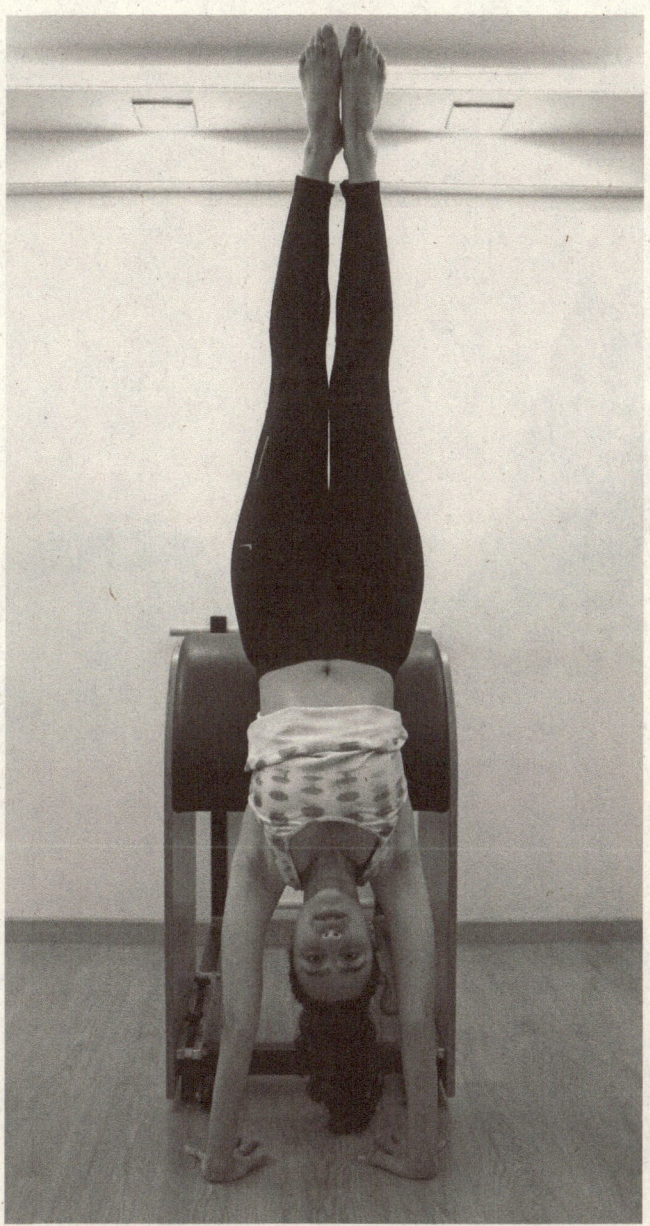

Pilates handstand on the Ladder Barrel.

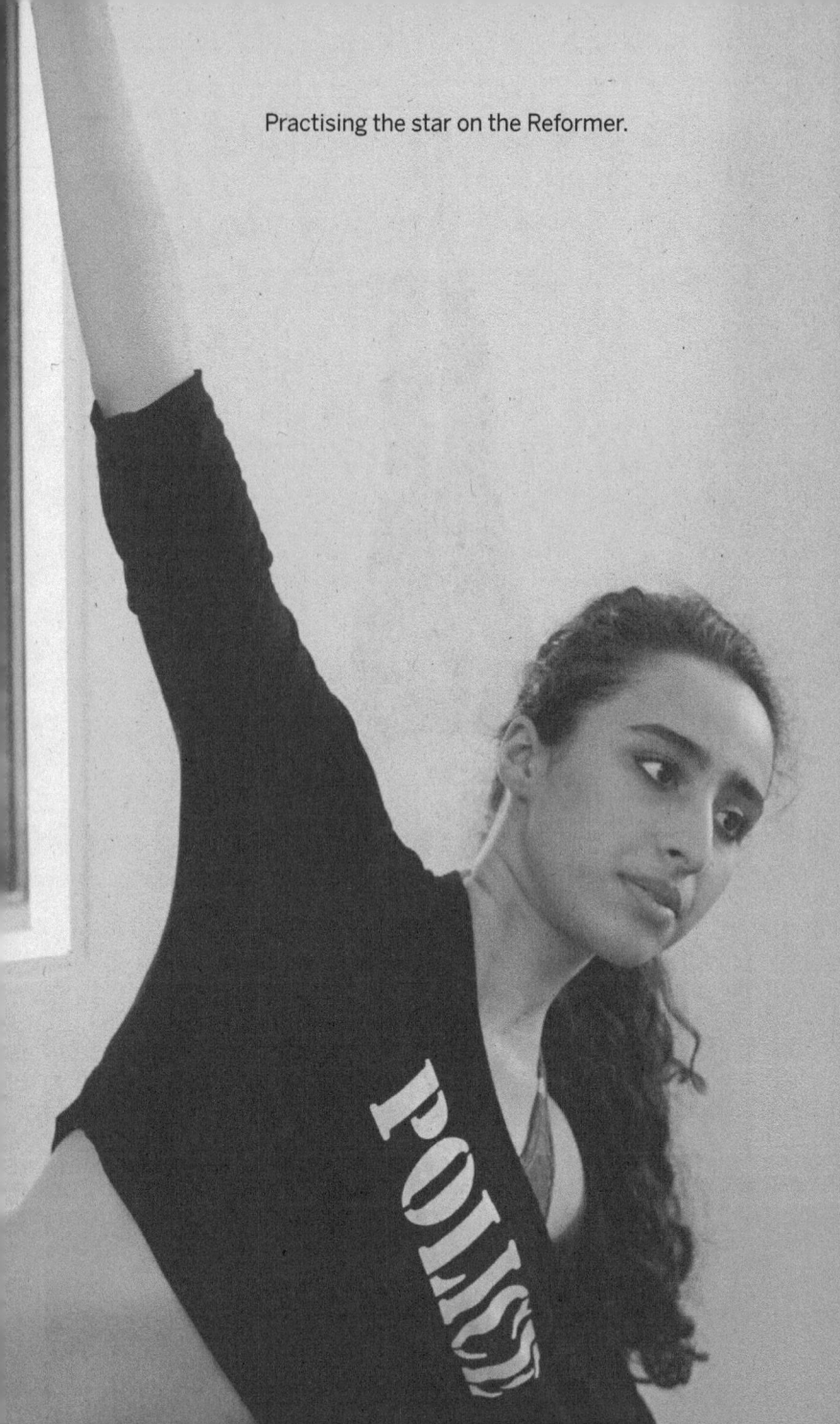

Practising the star on the Reformer.

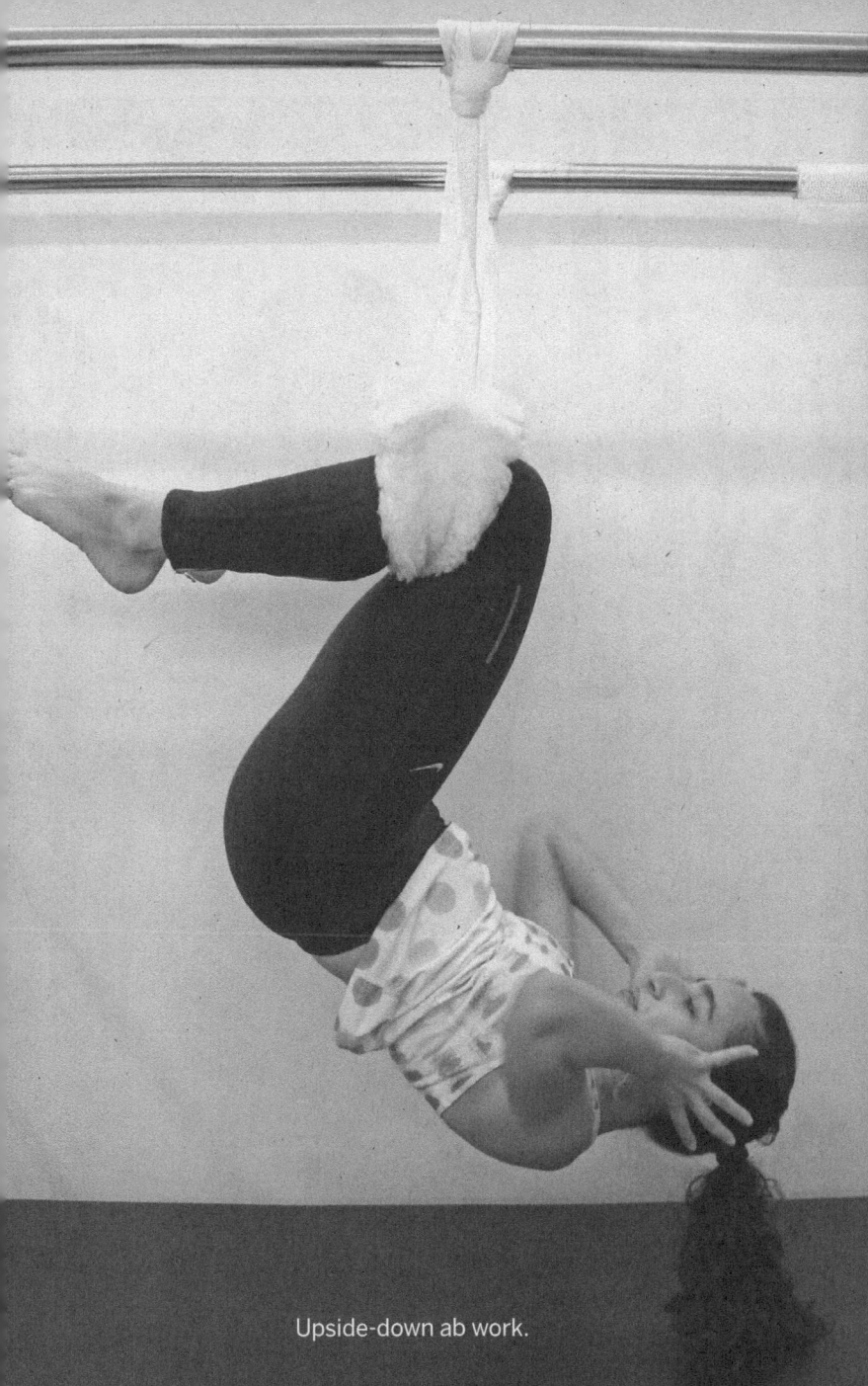

Upside-down ab work.

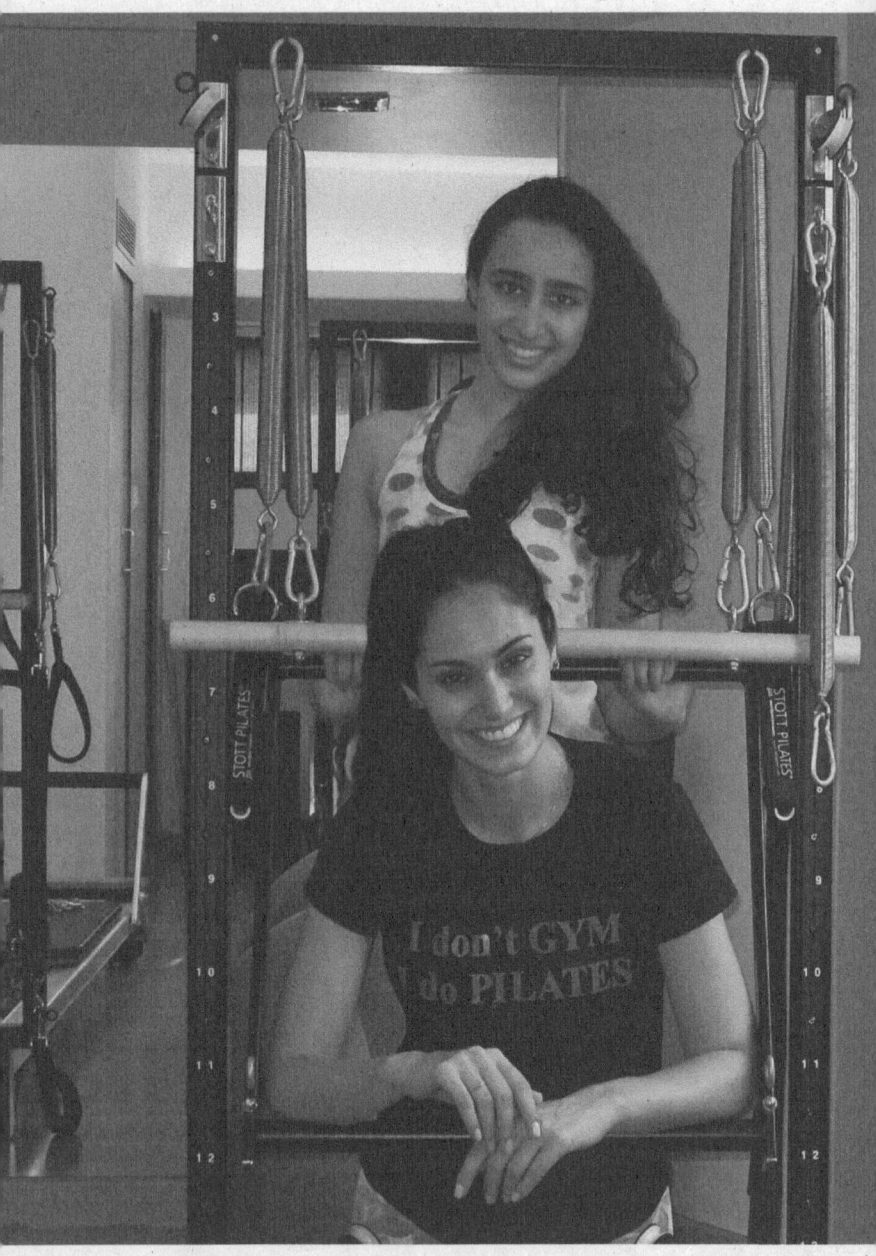
We don't gym, we do PILATES: Bruna Abdullah and Namrata.

- Abdominal crunches: 20 repetitions
- Abdominal side twist (working obliques): 20 repetitions (10 repetitions on each side)
- Back extension: 10 repetitions
- Stretches of all body parts: 5–10 minutes at the very least

All of the above should be done using the 3-set method. By the time you finish your training, you would have done almost 60 sets of various exercises, and spent approximately 90–120 minutes a day, 3 times a week.

Push-and-Pull Method, 3-set Routine: You should start with a weight with which you can do 12–15 repetitions in the first set—this acts as a kind of warm-up for that body part. Do approximately 10–12 repetitions of the second set, and the third would lead to muscle fatigue in approximately 8–10 repetitions. You should rest for about 1 or 2 minutes between sets—you can use this time to stretch the working muscle.

❖ **Day 1 (Monday) and Day 4 (Thursday)**
- Push-ups
- Flat chest press
- Incline chest press
- Decline chest press
- Pec fly
- Front shoulder raise
- Lateral shoulder raise

- Overhead press
- Tricep extension (overhead)
- Tricep kick-back
- Tricep press-down
- Abdominal exercise: Perform crunches (till you are fatigued). Ensure that your pelvis is stable and feet firmly grounded, with the knees bent while doing crunches. Do not use your lower-back muscles to come up into a crunch.
- Low back (back-extension exercises): 10 repetitions. Do not come higher than your pubic bone, i.e., ensure that your pubic bone is well grounded.
- Stretches: 5–10 minutes

By the time you complete your exercise routine, you would have done approximately 40 sets. The time expected to be taken for this routine would be approximately 75–90 minutes, twice a week.

❖ **Day 2 (Tuesday) and Day 5 (Friday)**
- Leg extension
- Leg curl
- Leg press
- Incline leg-press
- Calf raises
- Lat pulldown
- Mid-row

- Compound row
- Single-arm row
- Bicep curl
- Hammer curl
- Concentration curl
- Abdominal exercise: Perform crunches (till you are fatigued). Ensure that your pelvis is stable and feet are firmly grounded, with the knees bent while doing crunches. Do not use your lower-back muscles to come up into a crunch.
- Low back (back-extension exercises): Do not come higher than your pubic bone, i.e., ensure that your pubic bone is well grounded.
- Stretches: 5–10 minutes

By the time you complete your exercise routine, you would have done approximately 40 sets. The time expected to be taken for the above is approximately 75–90 minutes, twice a week. Remember that day 3 (Wednesday), day 6 (Saturday) and day 7 (Sunday) are rest/recovery days.

Of the two methods above, I personally prefer the push-and-pull method as I find it very effective in muscle activation. It provides great results.

Training to Muscle Failure: While exercising with weights, we usually tend to exercise with moderate to heavy weights. This set is completed without the muscle reaching complete failure. Here, the muscles feel worked out and then we do more sets and move to other body parts. This sort of workout is great for getting stronger and also for achieving reasonably bigger muscle mass.

In training to muscle failure, you train in such a way that you cannot do a single more repetition (30–40 repetitions). This way, you train to complete muscle fatigue, thus recruiting more muscle fibre and moving towards lean body mass.

However, in this sort of training, there is a huge demand on the mind and body and hence you could probably do this, say, 2–3 days a week, with at least a day's rest after each workout.

Tabata Intervals: This workout is designed to save time and simultaneously give a great strength-and-cardio workout. The routine comprises high-intensity interval training and consists of 20 seconds of high-intensity work followed by 10 seconds of rest, repeated 8 times. The time spent on this routine would be 4 minutes, but believe me, those 4 minutes would be very taxing on your cardiovascular system.

Dr Izumi Tabata's study showed that this 20-second-work-and-10-second-rest routine gives a great aerobic and anaerobic workout, improving cardiovascular output dramatically. This routine can be done in an actual sports environment, while running or swimming, or even by using your body weight.

Benefits of Strength Training

❖ Lifting weights makes one stronger, helps one with everyday activities and does not lead to 'bulking up'. In fact it helps one tone down, improves flexibility and makes one stronger.

❖ Nutrition is the key to any workout programme, so it is important to note that too much protein (more than 1 gm per 0.5 kg of body weight) is converted into fat and stored in the body, so do take a nutritionist's advice before starting your workout regime.

❖ Strength training increases a person's metabolic rate, i.e., there is an increase in the rate at which calories are burned as there is an increase in muscle. This consumes more energy. You will burn more calories all day long. For each pound of muscle, you will burn 35–50 calories daily. For example, if you gain 1.3 kg of muscle and burn 40 extra calories for each pound, you will burn 120 more calories per day or approximately 3600 calories per month, which equates to a loss of 4.5–5.4 kg in one year.

❖ Strength training can be done by women of all ages, even those 70 or 80 years of age, as it helps improve your functional life.

❖ It is said that strength training can increase spinal bone mineral density by 13 per cent in 6 months. Hence, it actually helps fight osteoporosis.

❖ Studies say that strength training can increase glucose utilization in the body by 23 per cent in 4 months, thereby reducing the risk of diabetes.

❖ A study mentions that strength-training exercises have a success rate of reducing lower-back pain in 80 per cent of the cases. Studies also indicate that strength training can ease arthritic pain and strengthen the joints.

❖ Strength training not only makes you a better athlete but also reduces the risk of injury.

Functional Training (Neuromotor Exercise):

The ACSM guidelines for functional training are:

❖ Neuromotor exercise (sometimes called 'functional fitness training') is recommended 3 days per week.

❖ Exercises should involve motor skills (balance, agility, coordination and gait), proprioceptive exercise training and multifaceted activities (t'ai chi and yoga) to improve physical function and prevent falls in older adults.

❖ About 20–30 minutes per day is appropriate for neuromotor exercise.

Some functional training routines that are easy to follow at home are given below:

❖ **Workout 1**
  - 50 Crunches
  - 25 Leg lifts
  - 50 Bicycles (lying on back)
  - 25 Squats
  - 15 Sumo squats (with weights—optional)
  - 50 Calf raises
  - 100 Arm circles (50 right and 50 left)
  - 15 Push-ups
  - 50 Jumping jacks

- Planking (1 minute)

Repeat the above 2–3 times. Please bear in mind that it is important to stretch well.

- ❖ **Workout 2**
  - 30 Jumping jacks
  - 5 Push-ups
  - 25 High knees
  - 7 Burpees
  - 10 Crunches
  - 7 Squats
  - 5 Push-ups
  - 10 Crunches
  - 5 Push-ups
  - 7 Squats
  - 30 Jumping jacks
  - Wall sit (1 minute)
  - 5 Push-ups
  - 25 High knees

Repeat the above 3–5 times. Please bear in mind that it is important to stretch very well.

- **Workout 3**
  - A combination strength-and-cardio workout can do wonders for your fitness level. It is a great way to

burn fat, increase muscle tone and improve endurance levels.

Strength and Cardio: 24 Minutes, Non-stop

❖ Full-body workout (with cardio) circuit: 24 minutes
❖ 1 set tempo, 2 seconds concentric and 4 seconds eccentric

You must reach muscle failure in 10–12 repetitions (so each exercise will be for one minute)

The circuit of squats, lunges, calf raises, push-ups, pec fly (on box), lat pull, mid-row, overhead shoulder (dumb-bell), tricep extension, bicep abdominal and back extension is to be done with a 45–60 second cardio burst after each exercise. For instance, you can run or skip on the spot or do burpees or mountain climbers or keep the treadmill on—say, at a 7.5 km speed—and jump on it, jog, and so on. The above routine is a great calorie buster as you are doing cardio and strength training almost non-stop for 24 minutes. The session will last approximately 24 minutes. Repeat twice if you are up to it. Remember that it is important to stretch well.

Flexibility Exercise/Stretching: The ACSM guidelines for flexibility and stretching are as follows:

❖ Adults should do flexibility exercises at least 2 or 3 days each week to improve their range of movements.
❖ Each stretch should be held for 10–30 seconds to the point of tightness or slight discomfort.

❖ Repeat each stretch 2–4 times, accumulating 60 seconds per stretch.

❖ Static, dynamic, ballistic and PNF stretches (mentioned in Chapter 3) are all effective.

❖ Flexibility exercises are most effective when the muscles are warm. Try light aerobic activity or a hot bath to warm up the muscles before stretching.

Why Stretch?

❖ It improves flexibility, reducing the chance of injury.

❖ Tight, stiff muscles limit the range of movements and, in some cases, can be a contributing factor to back and neck pain. Tight, stiff muscles cannot contract and relax efficiently, hence there is decreased performance and a lack of muscle movement control, leading to a loss of strength and power during physical activity.

❖ In a small percentage of cases, tight, stiff muscles can even have an effect on blood circulation. Good blood circulation is vitally important so that the muscles are able to receive adequate amounts of oxygen and nutrients. This can result in increased muscle fatigue and the ability to recover from strenuous exercise, impeding the muscle-repair process, which again can result in an increased chance of injury.

❖ As you age, your muscles and joints seem to get tighter and stiffer, which is part of the normal ageing process caused by a combination of physical degeneration and inactivity. Nevertheless, you must keep trying to improve your flexibility, especially if you are over 35. It improves athletic performance.

❖ It minimizes muscle soreness.

Besides the exercises mentioned above, there are many other ways to exercise and reach a great fitness level. I have listed two of them and explained them briefly below:

❖ **Pilates** is currently the buzzword for almost everyone in the showbiz industry, dancers as well as athletes, as it is very safe and of very low impact, which makes the risk of injury almost zero.

- Pilates was, in fact, one of the most favoured forms of exercise at the London Olympics in 2012 for almost all the participants.

- Pilates is almost 100 years old. It was a method of exercise developed by Joseph Pilates for injured soldiers during World War II. Due to the shortage of men during the war, it was imperative to have the injured soldiers back at the front line at the earliest, after their rehabilitation, of course. Joseph Pilates called it *contrology*, as all the exercises are done with utmost control by stabilizing the spine and working the muscles around it. He stressed the importance of being tension-free in an exercise position before starting an exercise.

- Joseph Pilates studied humans and their movement patterns and came to the conclusion that most movements are in the forward or flexion phase; hence the first few exercises he developed were more to do with trunk and hip flexion.

- Pilates was historically reformed for ballet and contemporary dancers. I often like to say that when you do Pilates you are preparing for war, but you will look like a ballet dancer. By this I mean that you will become extremely strong and flexible and enjoy great posture too.

- In Pilates, you are taught in detail about working the body through various planes: the sagittal (forward and backward movement); frontal (left to right; for example, side bends and lateral raises); and transverse (mainly rotational moves) planes, by following the 5 basic principles of Pilates. These include breathing, pelvic placement (neutral 'S' of the spine), ribcage placement, shoulder stability and neck (cervical), and head placement. These are the key to performing the exercise safely and efficiently. This is why we should follow the 5 principles:

  - *Breathing*: Proper breathing is extremely important due to the following reasons:

    - It gives extra oxygen to the working muscles and helps reduce stress, while simultaneously helping in the repair of microscopic tears in the muscles caused during the exercise.

    - Exhaling with pursed lips (with a bit of force) engages the transverse abdominal muscles (core) to form a corset, helping you to stabilize yourself before any movement takes place.

– Inhaling laterally and three-dimensionally keeps the core engaged. This breathing pattern enables the breath to go into the lower lobes of the lungs, reducing stress and increasing stamina. It is important to breathe into the back and sides of the ribcage when inhaling, and allowing the ribcage to relax while exhaling.

• *Pelvic Placement/Neutral 'S' of the Spine*: Being in the neutral 'S' of the spine helps you maintain the normal curve of the spine. The neutral 'S' is achieved when the front of the hip bones (anterior superior iliac spine) and the pubic bone are parallel to the floor (when you are lying on your back). Being in the neutral 'S' of the spine helps absorb the daily shocks that the body is subjected to; for instance, while walking or when wearing heels, etc.

• *Ribcage Placement*: The position of the ribcage affects the alignment of the thoracic (upper) spine. When lying on your back in a neutral position, the ribs should be resting gently on the mat—i.e., you should maintain the normal curve of the upper back. You should not lift the ribcage or push it into the mat. By doing this, you relax the stress in the ribcage and make exercise easier and stress-free.

• *Shoulder Stability*: Learn to stabilize the shoulder blades (scapulae) on the back of the ribcage by gently keeping your upper-back muscles engaged. As the shoulders have a lot of mobility due to a lack of direct bone attachment to the spine or to the ribcage, it is extremely important to emphasize this stability.

- *Head and Neck Placement*: It is important that your neck—i.e., the cervical spine—be in its natural curve, with the head above the shoulders when sitting, lying down and standing. You should feel a sense of lengthening around the neck region prior to exercise as this releases all the stress around the neck prior to and during exercise.

Further, Pilates comprises, by itself, a good workout routine, because of which there is no need to do anything else (except cardio). Like I mentioned before, Pilates is like preparing for war while looking like a ballet dancer. After all, it was initially meant for men fighting a war, but was then reformed for ballet dancers.

Doing Pilates 3 times a week (along with a good nutrition plan) is sufficient to achieve your fitness goal. Each session of Pilates normally lasts approximately 50 minutes or so. Joseph Pilates believed it took 10 sessions to feel the difference, 20 sessions to see the difference and 30 sessions to have a brand-new body.

You can also go to the gym and lift weights—Pilates will actually enhance the experience. It teaches you about control, stability and precise movement.

Benefits of Pilates

As I have mentioned before, Pilates is beneficial for general fitness, specific health conditions and, most of all, for your overall well-being. It does the following:

- Improves and strengthens the core (abs)
- Improves muscle tone and flexibility
- Improves your posture
- Complements training for athletes
- Facilitates injury prevention and physical rehabilitation
- Builds better balance and coordination, particularly for the elderly
- Offers a safe and excellent form of exercise for women in the antenatal and postnatal stages
- Helps maintain—and even improves—bone density
- Develops the function and efficiency of the lungs with improvement in circulation
- Offers a safe and beneficial form of exercise for a wide range of medical conditions including scoliosis, osteoporosis, arthritis and multiple sclerosis
- Relieves stress and tension and promotes a feeling of well-being
- Makes you look and feel better

There are many Pilates DVDs available in the market which can help you achieve a fair level of fitness. However, it would be great to have an experienced trainer come home or, better still, to go to a good Pilates studio which has good trainers. This can help you achieve a good level of fitness.

❖ **Simulated Altitude Training:** About 10–15 years after the 1964 Mexico Olympics, scientists found that training at high altitudes for a period of time helped international athletes improve their performance levels drastically. Altitude training caused physiological changes in their bodies and, among other things, buffered the build-up of lactic acid, allowing the athletes to sustain their performance at the topmost level of their game for a longer period of time, especially at sea level. Besides improving athletic performance, altitude training provides many other benefits to an individual. Only recently has the outside world started understanding and using this method of training for weight loss, diabetes control, asthma treatment, and so on.

Simulated altitude training can be done individually by using a mask system, or it can be done in a room which is set at a simulated altitude of 2800 metres or more—the idea being to basically simulate the oxygen levels found at those heights.

Now, allow me to explain simulated altitude training and how it works. At sea level, the oxygen level in your blood is between 96 and 99 per cent, and the oxygen level in the air is 20.9 per cent. When you exercise at sea level, the oxygen levels in your blood do not drop below 96 per cent, however hard you train, even though there is an increase in your heart rate and breathing pattern. Due to this, there is an increase in the oxygen supply in the blood and consequently to your working muscles.

When you exercise (mainly cardiovascular training) in low-oxygen air, i.e., at approximately 2700 metres or higher (meaning, when there is 15 per cent oxygen or lower), there is an increase in your heart rate and breathing pattern and there is an attempt to get more oxygen into your blood.

Due to this, there is an increase in your metabolic rate, which helps you burn almost 200 per cent more calories in the same number of minutes you would spend training at sea level. Weight loss is drastically increased if you train at a simulated altitude. But you must remember that nothing happens without good nutrition.

In a simulated altitude-training room, you can exercise on the treadmill, elliptical trainer, cycle, functional training, etc. For more information on simulated altitude-training, you can contact the fitness centres around your residence.

I hope I have been able to give you some insight into improving your fitness through the various methods listed to help you reach your fitness goals. The above details will help you understand different forms of exercising and also make you more aware of what you are doing.

It is important for you to know why you are exercising and train accordingly: Is it for a competition, or is it for general fitness? Be realistic about your goals. Don't be desperate to achieve them too quickly as fitness is not a one-time fling—it is a way of life—and it will take some time for you to achieve your fitness goals. But once you are there, it is the best feeling ever.

7

TALKING ABOUT FOOD

I am now going to tell you something which is by far the most important tool in your fitness goals: nutrition. You have to be aware that without good nutrition, you are not going to reach your fitness goals and attain a dream body. Nutrition constitutes 70–80 per cent of your fitness regime and hence it is important to have at least a working knowledge of it.

Before you start your fitness journey, it is essential to have your doctor's clearance that indicates that you are fit enough to exercise. The next step is to go to a nutritionist and plan your food intake depending on the kind of training you are planning to go in for. Some of the parameters that you should check prior to starting your fitness regime are weight, BMI (body mass index), body fat and BMR (basal metabolic rate).

Here are some guidelines as to what would be a close-to-ideal reading of the above. You can check this at home on your own:

❖ **Weight**: Ideal body weight can be measured as under:

Ideal Body Weight (kg) = Height (cm) − 100

For example, if your height is 162.5 cm, then your ideal body weight (kg) would be:

162.5 − 100 = 62.5 kg

However, it is important to remember that the above figure has to be seen together with −5 range for women and a +5 range for men.

Therefore:

Ideal body weight for women is between 57.5 and 62.5 kg

Ideal body weight for men is between 62.5 and 67.5 kg

❖ **BMI:** This is measured as under:

BMI = kg/sq. of height in metres

For example, if a person is 87 kg and his height is 162.5 cm, then the BMI will be calculated as under:

= 87 kg/sq. of height in metres (1.625 metre)

= 87 kg/2.64

= 32.95

Following are the figures to be kept in mind for the required BMI:

< 19   : Underweight

19–25   : Normal

25–30   : Grade 1 Obesity

30–40   : Grade 2 Obesity

> 40   : Grade 3 Obesity (morbid obesity)

❖ **Waist-to-Hip Ratio:** Here is an example of how this is to be calculated. If one's waist is 24 inches and the hips are 36 inches, then the waist-to-hip ratio is = 24/36 = 0.66.

These are the ideal required specifications you can keep in mind:

Women   : < 0.85

Men   : < 0.90

❖ **BMR:** This means the number of calories expended in a day doing daily chores, resting, and so on.

The way to calculate your BMR (as per the YMCA method), depending on whether you are male or female, is as under:

Male: 66 + (12.7 x height [inches]) + (6.23 x weight [lbs]) − (6.8 x age)

Example. : 66 + (12.7 x 71) + (6.23 x 160) − (6.8 x 45) = − (66 + 901.7) + (996.8) − (306) = 1658.5 kcal per day

Female: 665 + (4.7 x height [inches]) + (4.35 x weight ([lbs]) − (4.7 x age)

Eg. : 665 + (4.7 x 63) + (4.35 x 132) − (4.7 x 45)

= 665 + 296.1 + 574.2 − 211.5 = 1323.8 kcal per day

You can calculate the Resting Metabolic Rate (RMR or BMR) by the above formulae, but as per the YMCA, it is necessary to add an activity factor.

Hence, as per the YMCA:

❖ If your lifestyle leads you to sit most of the time (studying, reading, watching TV): Add 20 per cent to your BMR

❖ If you engage in light activity (teaching, etc.): Add 30 per cent to your BMR.

❖ If you spend most of your time moving around and possibly lifting light objects (cooking, light workouts, etc.): Add 40 per cent to your BMR.

❖ If you move heavy objects, play professional sports, do heavy workouts, or engage in hard manual work: Add 50 per cent to your BMR.

Hence, you can calculate the required calories in your food intake. For example, if a woman spent 1323.8 calories in a day, add 50 per cent, as per the above calculations (due to heavy workouts, etc.), her calorie intake should be 1323.8 + 661.9 = 1985.7 kcal per day to maintain her weight. However, if she wants to lose weight, then she should opt for a diet that is approximately 500 kcal less than the above, i.e., 1985.7 − 500 = 1485.7 kcal per day. This means that she would consume 500 × 7 days = 3500 calories, i.e., she would end up losing 1 kg per week, which is a safe way to lose weight.

Please do not consume less than 1200 kcal per day, as then the nutritional value will reduce dramatically.

❖ **Body Fat (Percentage):** Body fat essentially means the amount of fat in your body. If you are 68 kg, and your body fat is 20 per cent, then your body fat is 13.6 kg, and the balance is lean body mass, i.e., muscle, organs, bone, blood, etc.

Body Fat Guidelines from the American Council on Exercise

Classification	% Fat (Women)	% Fat (Men)
Essential Fat	10–12	2–4
Athletes	14–20	6–13
Fitness	21–24	14–17
Acceptable	25–31	18–25
Obese	32+	25+

I personally feel that the most important element above is body fat, as this gives you a true indication of how much fat you have in your body. BMR would help a nutritionist plan her/his nutrition plan according to the calories expended by an individual. The other parameters really depend a lot on your frame or body structure.

Now, let me try and explain to you a little about the foods available to us. These macronutrients are essentially broken up into carbohydrates, fats and proteins; the ratio in which they are to be taken per day depends on the age of the person concerned.

Up to the age of 18, a person requires the following approximate amount of nutrients:

Carbohydrates: 45–65 per cent
Proteins: 20–30 per cent
Fats: 30-40 per cent

For adults, however, there is a slight difference:

Carbohydrates: 45–65 per cent
Proteins: 10–35 per cent
Fats: 20–35 per cent

Before we go into details of the macronutrients, we should know a little about the food values:

Carbohydrates: 1 gm = 4 calories
Proteins: 1 gm = 4 calories
Fats: 1 gm = 9 calories

HOW TO CALCULATE THE PERCENTAGE VALUES OF FOOD ITEMS?

A general healthy-eating guideline is to get 60 per cent of your calories from carbohydrates, 20 per cent from proteins and 20 per cent from fats. The American Heart Association recommends eating 20–30 per cent fats on a daily basis. You should never have a meal that has more than 30 per cent fat.

To calculate percentage values of various foods, work out the details based on the calculation below:

For instance, if a food is listed as having 170 calories and is said to contain 10 gm total fats, 6 gm proteins and 14 gm carbohydrates, then the total percentage of each of these would be as under:

Multiply the grams with the calories per gm as listed above:

Carbohydrates: 14 gm x 4 calories per gm = 56 calories
Proteins: 6 gm x 4 calories per gm = 24 calories
Fats: 10 gms x 9 calories per gm = 90 calories

Total calories = 170 calories

Now, divide the calories of each of the nutrients by the total number of calories:

Carbohydrate: 56/170 = 33 per cent
Protein: 24/170 = 14 per cent
Fat: 90/170 = 53 per cent

From the above calculation, you can see that there is too much fat percentage in your food. Hence, whenever you eat something, make sure you check how much fat it contains. It's a good way to know how good or bad your diet is. You can do it a couple of times just so that you become more aware about things that aren't so great and things that are pretty good.

Let us speak a little about each of these macronutrients:

Carbohydrates

Carbohydrates are the best source of fuel. A diet should ideally consist of complex carbohydrates (which contain nutrients and fibre) as against simple carbohydrates (which are found in sugar and sweets). Here, I list some of the simple carbohydrates (also known as simple sugars) and complex carbohydrates (also known as starch) for your guidance:

Simple carbohydrates: These are essentially foods which have a high glycemic index. They are found in sugar and sweets. If you are having an ice cream, then you are consuming simple carbohydrates. Simple sugars are found in food in its natural form, and hence it is better to get simple sugars from natural foods like milk, fruit, and so on.

Complex carbohydrates: These are essentially foods which have a low glycemic index; for example, bread, pasta, rice, etc.

Glycemic Index: This is a number that gives us information about the effect of a particular food on your blood-sugar levels. In this case, 100 means pure glucose (simple carbohydrates). If you have a lower reading, it indicates complex carbohydrates.

Therefore, it is better to have foods with a low glycemic index as these are absorbed slowly into the blood stream, thereby giving energy to the person over a longer period of time. Here is a list of some foods with good and bad carbohydrates, according to the Harvard School of Public Health:

Fruit

- *Good carbs*: Apples, pears, oranges, lemons, grapes, cherries, peaches, apricots, plums, kiwis, papayas, mangoes, melons, strawberries
- *Bad carbs*: Raisins, fruit juice

Nuts

- *Good carbs*: Almonds, walnuts, sesame seeds, sunflower seeds, hazelnuts, Brazil nuts, pecans, macadamia nuts
- Bad carbs: Honey-roasted nuts, any nuts coated with sugar

Legumes

- *Good carbs*: Peanuts, cashew nuts, peas (if eaten in moderate quantity), black beans (if eaten in moderate quantity), rajma, chickpeas
- *Bad carbs*: Any of the sweetened variety

Beverages

- *Good carbs*: Water, tea, coffee, wine
- *Bad carbs*: Soda, beer, juice, sweet tea

Grains

- *Good carbs*: Wholewheat, brown rice, sprouted grains, oats, wholegrain pasta
- *Bad carbs*: White rice or flour or bread, pasta, sweetened foods like cakes and muffins

Vegetables

- *Good carbs*: Leafy vegetables, cauliflower, broccoli, cabbages, cucumbers, tomatoes
- *Bad carbs*: Potatoes

Proteins

They are the structural components of all body tissue and are essential for growth, maintenance and repair. Protein is not a fuel source, but is very important for hormones, etc. An increased intake of proteins can cause liver and kidney damage as well as too much body fat and a drastic reduction in calcium.

How much protein is required per day?

- Kids can do with 1 gm of protein per kg of body weight.
- Adults need protein depending on their workload in a day. For example, a sedentary adult can get away with 1–1.2 gm of protein per kg of body weight, while an adult involved in heavy training needs up to 1.7 gm of protein per kg of body fat.

In percentage terms, a sedentary adult would need 12 per cent of protein per day, while an adult involved in heavy training needs up to 18–24 per cent protein.

Here is a list of proteins:
- *Meat*: Lamb, goat
- *Seafood*: Anchovies, groupers, kingfish, mackerel, salmon, sardines, swordfish, trout, tuna, clams, crabs, lobsters, prawns, oysters, shrimps
- *Poultry and eggs*: Chicken, duck, goose, turkey; chicken eggs, duck eggs
- *Beans and peas*: Black beans, chickpeas (garbanzo beans), falafel, kidney beans, lentils, soybeans, tofu, white beans

- *Nuts and seeds*: Almonds, cashew nuts, hazelnuts, mixed nuts, peanuts, pistachios, pumpkin seeds, sesame seeds, sunflower seeds, walnuts

Fats

Fats are a source of fuel and are carriers of various vitamins such as A, D, E and K. We all need a certain amount of fat, though an overdose of them can cause heart disease and diabetes. There are various types of fats in your food and they are listed below:

- *Monosaturated fats*: Olive oil, canola oil—these are the best options
- *Polyunsaturated fats*: Fish oils, vegetable oils
- *Saturated fats*: Butter, margarine
- *Trans-fatty acids*: These raise the cholesterol and increase the risk of heart disease

Here is a short list of fats:

- *Good fats*: Olive oil, soybean oil, canola oil, sunflower oil
- *Bad fats*: Mayonnaise, packaged snacks, peanut butter, fried food, croissants, sausages, cream

Here are some healthy alternatives for bad fats:

Fats to Avoid	Alternatives
Whole egg	Egg white
Whole milk	Skimmed milk
Whipped cream	Skim-milk cream

Let me give you a little insight on how you should plan your menu for the day. The number of calories you consume in a day depends on the activities you do in a day and your age. For a woman and/or an older adult leading a sedentary lifestyle, consuming approximately 1600–1700 calories would be adequate per day. A child, teenage girl, active woman and many sedentary men would need up to approximately 2000–2200 calories per day. A teenage boy, active men and very active women would need approximately 2700–2800 calories per day.

Here is some information on the recommended per-day servings of the different food types:

- **Water:** This is the most important. Have at least 8–10 glasses of water a day, keeping in mind that each glass should be approximately 250 ml. Water should be had before, during and after exercise, so as to replace the fluids lost during the process. Water also energizes the body.

- **Fats:** These should be used very sparingly. But it is important to include fats for a balanced diet.

- **Dairy Products:** Have at least 2–4 servings of dairy products in a day. But choose products that are low in fat percentage.

- **Vegetables:** Have at least 3–5 servings a day. A good idea would be to have dark leafy vegetables, which are better and richer in nutrients than say, iceberg lettuce. While cooking vegetables it is better to steam or stir-fry them so as to minimize the loss of vitamins and minerals.

- **Fruit:** A minimum of 2–4 servings a day is good.

- **Grains:** Have 6–11 servings a day. Try to have wholegrain bread, brown rice and wholewheat pasta, as these are high in fibre. Also, eating fibre helps stabilize blood sugar, keeps you satisfied for a longer time and helps you avoid food cravings.

- **Meat:** Have 2–3 servings of meat.

I hope I have been able to give you an idea of your nutrition plan in a day. However, I recommend that for the best results, visit a nutritionist who can specifically guide you to help you reach your fitness goals.

8

BALANCE: PUTTING IT ALL TOGETHER

J ust like everything else in life, having a balanced exercise regime and diet is essential. A good diet and exercise routine go hand in hand—there is little or no point doing one without the other. Both are basic things we need to do for ourselves. We deserve to give ourselves nutritious food that not only makes us look good but also keeps us healthy. We also deserve a good exercise regime that increases our strength, makes us feel good and strong, flexible and fit.

You must remember that getting fit, losing weight and making a healthy diet a part of your lifestyle is not something that will happen overnight. Losing weight and, for some of you, even gaining 'good weight', and getting your dream body is something that requires time and dedication. You've got to be focused, stay on the right path and make long-lasting changes in your routine. If you manage to strike a good balance in your life, you will find that the results are amazing and long-lasting. Not only will you look great but you will also feel great about yourself. I strongly believe that you control your own destiny, and taking care of your health from a young age will pay off in the future. Commit yourself to yourself! You deserve that.

You have to strike a balance in your life. The first and most important thing to do is to fix your diet. This does not mean that you have to starve or refrain from eating the things you like—it only means eating enough of the good things, and having unhealthy food in moderation. According to me, eating healthy doesn't mean you are on a diet, it's simply eating right—the way it should be. Your body needs all the nutrients and enough energy to get through the day. It basically means getting used to a better, healthier lifestyle. Once you cut down on unhealthy food and incorporate nutritious food into your diet, you will not want to go back to eating unhealthy as you will see the difference in your body. You will feel lighter and more energized, you will look fresher and feel more positive.

The next thing to do is to figure out which fitness regime you like and what you enjoy doing. I have already mentioned quite a few fun activities you could do. You could go the traditional way and join a gym, you could start with skipping and easy-to-do exercises at home, or you could join a dance class, go cycling, or even horse riding. Doing them all will give you a taste of each, and you'll also enjoy each activity more. You could do dance classes twice a week, go cycling once a week, run once a week, and go swimming or horse riding another day. Be sure to include some sort of strength training.

What you must remember is that fitness is not about having a six-pack or a muscular body, nor is it about being thin and skinny. Being fit is much more than that. Fitness includes various aspects such as flexibility, stamina, strength, great energy levels, endurance and a complete sense of well-being. It is more of a holistic term, and is not just about appearance—it is about what is going on inside your body. The heart should perform to its full potential, lung capacity should be good and high, and your muscles should not only be strong but also flexible.

Unfortunately, today, in our visual world, people have forgotten about real fitness and have drifted more towards what looks good. Different 'health' and 'fitness' products are being sold the world over to make you 'fit'. Unfortunately, the reality is that these products may not actually be good for you. You need to be aware of what is right for you and what is not. Any unnatural way of getting 'fit' means that you are *not* getting fit but perhaps only losing weight, which is an extremely small aspect of fitness. In the long run, these unnatural ways of losing weight could actually be more harmful, and you will eventually put on more weight over time—it might take a few months or a year, but you will.

Today, due to the widespread influence of film stars and models, many of us want to achieve a great body, and we want it quick, which is not only unnatural but also very harmful for the body. Achieving 'that look' quickly is drastic—it will not help you and will cause more harm than good. So why put your body through that? Why not be a little focused, give yourself some time, and do it the right way? There is no better feeling than working out sincerely and regularly and achieving your fitness goals. Going about the process naturally and correctly means that you will not only lose weight but also get stronger and more flexible, thereby moving towards true fitness. Isn't that better? Isn't that what we want? Being truly fit? That is the most important thing.

A very dear client of mine, singer and actor Manasi Scott—who, according to me, is extremely beautiful and has one of the most lovely voices I have ever heard—is a great example of how to believe in yourself and achieve true fitness. Manasi's goal has never been to become thin or skinny; she has always aimed at being fit, strong and flexible. She is one person who seems to have clearly understood the true meaning of fitness. Manasi's routine with me comprises altitude training and Pilates thrice a week. This is just about an hour and a half, 3 times a week, that she dedicates to me. Though she has a busy schedule and a hectic life, she tries her best to make it for these sessions. She travels an hour to get to my studio and an hour to go back, but she is there. On days that she cannot make it, she does some exercises at home and tries to go for a run outdoors. I help Manasi work her body inside out. This means that we are not only focusing on doing harder, tougher exercises but also relaxing and soothing exercises that may not be as challenging, but definitely work the muscles deeply and relax the mind. Manasi eats well and has her meals on time. She does not starve herself to lose weight, but ensures that she gets all the necessary nutrients. Sometimes, we go outdoors and go horse riding together, which again is a great way to work out, de-stress and mix things up a bit. This keeps Manasi's workout interesting. Due to her inherent dedication and focus—not only now, but right from a young age—Manasi is stronger than most teenagers and more flexible too. She never gives up, and if her schedule ever goes for a toss, she tries her best to do some form of exercise and gets back on track as soon as possible. What you must learn is to strike the right balance between exercise, work and food. You should give your body enough time, and your mind too, so that as you grow older, it becomes much easier for you to stay fit and follow a healthy routine. This way you will always be 18 till you die.

It is a general belief that girls who are skinny and guys who are muscular are fit and thus do not need to work out. Well, maybe we should challenge a skinny girl to do 5 push-ups properly or to run 400 metres without being unreasonably breathless at the end of it, or to simply touch her toes and touch her head to her knee to judge how truly fit she is. If a girl on the slightly heavier side can do these things, I would say she is much fitter than the skinny girl. As I have said quite a few times, and can't stress its importance enough, fitness is *not* measured by how thin you are, but by how strong and flexible you are, the stamina you have, your energy levels, and other such factors.

While deciding your fitness goals, it is extremely important to look at the overall fitness benefits. You want to think about getting strong, lean, flexible, faster—and more fit. Set a goal that is smart, time-effective and time-bound.

Before you start your exercise regime, you must remember that doing more does not mean that you are doing better. Your workout should be effective, not strenuous. It should challenge you enough, but not cause unnecessary aches and pains in the body. I usually tell my clients that they do not need more than one hour of exercise a day. If you use this one hour well, you will get better benefits than exercising for hours daily, as your body will only overwork itself and get fatigued. Overdoing it can also cause strains, sprains or other injuries. What you must ensure is that you give your body one day of complete rest. Just as you get the weekend off from work or college to give your mind a break, you require the same for your body. Take a break and relax and rest your body.

Before setting out on the exercise regime of your choice, remember to wear the correct gear for it—the correct shoes and clothes. For example, ensure that you wear running shoes for running and the correct football shoes while playing football, as these are not interchangeable. Similarly, if you are going for a jazz dance class, it is advisable to wear jazz shoes or sneakers as these are better for your feet when you dance. Also, wear comfortable clothes that allow freedom of movement. You cannot possibly wear jeans and work out. Ensure that you wear the correct bra. Having the correct size and type of bra for your workout is necessary. Wear a good-quality sports bra; most shops stock sports bras depending on the impact of the sport you intend to practise. For example, for high-impact sports such as running and jumping, it is advisable to wear a sports bra made for high-impact training. Some sports or workout forms that you choose may require special protective gear such as helmets for horse riding or cycling, knee pads while skating, and the like. Ensure that you invest in them as they are for your own safety.

Before you start your exercise regime, remember to do a warm-up. Your warm-up should cover all the muscles that you are going to be working during your routine. It should be a dynamic warm-up of each and every major muscle group in the body as this will help prevent injuries and unnecessary wear and tear. When you practise exercises such as Pilates or yoga, a warm-up will be naturally incorporated into your routine, but gym-goers may sometimes forget how important a warm-up is. This negligence can result in aches and pains that can easily be avoided. A good warm-up usually lasts anywhere between 5 and 15 minutes, and is a must-do. Arm circles, walking for a few minutes, skipping or leg swings can be a part of your warm-up routine.

At the end of your workout, you have to do a cool-down, which usually means slowing down and relaxing the body. For instance, if you had been running, you should slow down to a jog and then to a walk. You must not just stop and leave. You must also stretch well. Stretch safely and slowly. Ballistic stretches, where you bounce the body, are not needed. Stretching helps relax and gives shape to the body. It also helps prevent injuries, which is crucial as it comes in the way of your fitness goals. You will feel more energetic and recover faster after a workout.

Basically, all you have to do is, do it 'right'. First, find the right activity, an activity you enjoy so that you do not stop halfway, which keeps you interested so that you are never bored, and which challenges you enough so that you are always striving to achieve more. There are so many things that you can do, from kickboxing to aerobics, cycling, running, skating, swimming, basketball, gymnastics, Pilates and dancing. With the variety and options out there, you will definitely find something you enjoy. Second, put on the correct gear and use the correct equipment for the activity of your choice. The equipment should be well maintained and dynamically correct. The gear you wear should be protective and comfortable. Third, you must only do the activity in the right doses. It is not necessary to work out for hours. You cannot do the same activity all day. Do not overwork and stress your muscles and joints. Train smart and train efficiently. Exercising too much in any form can cause fatigue and muscle exhaustion, lead to injury and may result in your becoming uninterested in the exercise quickly. You have to find the correct balance in your routine and get enough exercise and physical activity, but not too much. Do these few things correctly and you will be on the correct path.

Eating healthy and exercising regularly are two sides of the same coin. You are not going to get all the desired benefits of eating healthy without exercising, or all the benefits of exercising without eating healthy. If you do not eat well, do not eat the right amount, or undereat, you will not have enough energy to work out. Similarly, if you do not exercise, you could run the risk of developing high cholesterol or other such conditions. Similarly, overtraining or overeating can be harmful. Overtraining can lead to injuries and will add little or no added benefit to your regular regime. Overeating leads to excessive calorie intake, which leads to weight gain and a heavy feeling overall.

Finding a way to strike a good balance between food intake and exercise can be a challenge. In the case of losing weight, it is all about being able to take in fewer calories than you burn. If you have been sweating it out and training hard, but have not seen the weighing scale budge, it is probably because you are taking in more calories than you are burning. Here is where you have to stop, rethink your goals and adjust not only your exercise routine but also your diet. You have to be able to eat less than the number of calories you work off through the day in order to lose weight. If you are trying to maintain your weight and not put on any, then naturally the calories consumed should equal the calories burned. Every year, a million people make resolutions to take care of their health, eat healthy and lose weight. Not many end up sticking to their resolutions. If you are one of those people who have lost their way, now is the time to find the right path again. It is time to combine a healthy diet and fitness regime to get optimal results and acquire your dream body.

The simple principle behind weight loss is to burn more calories than you eat. It is really a great experience to be able to find that right balance between what you consume in your day-to-day diet and the amount you exercise. So if you eat 1200 calories, you must burn 1700 calories in the course of your daily activities so as to see a change on the weighing scale. If your diet is great, even a little increase in your regular exercise regime will get the scales moving. Similarly, a good exercise regime combined with an unhealthy diet will not really be beneficial, but a little improvement in your diet will do wonders for your body.

Counting the number of calories you eat can be a bit tricky, so getting the advice of dieticians or learning to cook dishes that are calorie-friendly are great ways to start. Nowadays, it is easy to find tasty, nutritious recipes online. You can look up breakfast, lunch or dinner options, replete with all the ingredients you like, and you could also discover new ideas or recipes you have not thought of making before. Even snacks are important, and making healthy ones is essential. Some of my favourite snacks are hummus with pita bread, bruschetta with very little olive oil, and fruit. In general, for women, a standard weight-loss diet usually consists of around a 1400-calorie intake a day. This, of course, may vary based on how active you are and certain other factors such as hormones, age, etc. What you eat is one of the key factors to losing weight. I do not believe in going on extreme diets, starving yourself, or any other drastic measures, as all of these are temporary and not long-lasting. You must follow a sustainable, healthy diet that will stay with you for a long time. It is about changing your eating habits for good, and that takes just a little time to get used to. You must be patient.

Eat a balanced diet and take in all the nutrients. Ensure that your diet comprises plenty of fruit and vegetables. Try consuming low-fat dairy products instead of the full-fat options. In case of sweet cravings, try substituting regular chocolate with dark chocolate. Another thing you can do to get rid of a sweet craving is to put some grapes in the freezer for 10 minutes and then eat them. They are pretty yummy and also help to get rid of the craving. Try and eat smaller meals at regular intervals. Have a good breakfast, lunch and dinner but also eat in between these meals as being on an empty stomach for too long is not good either. Eating well is an art that may initially feel difficult to master, but is the easiest to follow in the long run. It becomes a way of life.

When thinking about losing weight, think also about toning and sculpting the body. Your exercise regime should consist of a certain number of cardiovascular exercises, and toning and strength-training exercises. It may not always be possible to hit the gym, but there are lots of other things that you can do at home. Do mat-work exercises, skip, use the hula hoop, or do household work, as even these things can help you burn calories. Climb the stairs instead of using the elevator, walk short distances, get up and stroll to your co-workers' desks when you need to speak with them. These small, daily activities can make a big difference.

An ideal workout plan is one where you work out 4–5 days a week for 30–60 minutes, although this also depends on what sort of workout plan you decide to take up. You should do a good mix of cardiovascular exercises and strength-training exercises to get the best results. Cardio exercises build your stamina and endurance and burn some serious calories, while strength-training exercises build lean body mass, and sculpt and tone the body. Lean muscle helps burn fat, and the more lean muscle you have, the more calories your body will naturally burn. Strength-training exercises could include simple weight-training, for which you could also use your own body weight or do Pilates. My favourite regime comprises altitude training and Pilates. I practise Pilates about thrice a week, and use the simulated altitude-training room for 30 minutes, 3–4 times a week. I find this effective as even in the short duration of about an hour, I am able to get in strength as well as cardio exercises and can see the difference in my body. Whenever you start any workout regime, start realistically; you cannot expect to climb Mount Everest in one day. Start slow and steady, and gradually increase your strength, flexibility and endurance. You will be pleasantly surprised by what you can achieve by sticking to your regimen and training smart.

Another aspect—which, according to me, is an extremely important aspect—is your attitude towards yourself and your regime. If you enjoy the journey to a healthy fitness regime, you are sure to achieve your goals. My number one rule at the studio is to keep smiling. This not only makes me feel good but also motivates me to do better. Also, no one wants to see a grumpy face. Yes, achieving your goal may take time, but with dedication and focus you will get there. Do not be disheartened when you look at celebrities' bodies and see them seemingly achieve their goal in no time; you want to get more fit naturally, and in a healthy manner. Celebrities' jobs demand perfect bodies, and they need to be able to visually fit a role in the shortest amount of time. But you have the liberty to achieve your goals patiently and correctly. When you are happy with what you are doing, doing it becomes easy. That is why I advise you to choose a regime you enjoy, so that it is more of a stress buster than a stress creator. It should be something that makes you happy while you are at it, and de-stresses you. Just never, ever, ever give up! You can do it! All you need is some time and dedication.

When you manage to strike a balance, you will find yourself achieving your fitness goals in no time. Nothing will stop you, and you will have the power and positive energy to take you through the entire journey. I believe that if you have a difficulty and want better results, you should consult a professional as they can guide you properly. A well-qualified personal trainer or coach will know exactly what you need when she/he meets you and will be able to train you accordingly. The workout will then be customized to your body type and everything will be fine-tuned for you.

No obstacle is too hard to cross and no goal is too hard to attain. Go for it with all your heart and you will be there in no time. As I often say: Train smart!

9

HOLIDAY: EXERCISES FOR WHEN YOU ARE ON HOLIDAY

Exercise on a holiday?! What? No way! I think this is what most people would say. But, really, it is not such a big deal to keep your exercise regimen going while you are on vacation. It could actually be exciting, different—and interesting. Imagine running on the beach in Brazil or Hawaii, or going to Hyde Park in London for a jog, horse riding in the hills, or swimming in the beautiful Mediterranean Sea. Doesn't sound all that bad now, does it?

You do get out of the city at some point for some reason or another—a college or work-related trip, or simply a vacation—but this should not stop you from continuing your fitness routine, staying active and getting stronger. Yes, your normal conveniences and logistics may get a bit messed up, you may not have access to a gym, you may not be able to prepare your own meals, you may need to change your sleeping pattern—but nothing should stop you from continuing on your fitness path. Regardless of where you are, there is still a lot you can do. You can take a day to settle into the new place and figure out what's nearby and what's happening, but day 2 onwards you should get right back on track. Going on a vacation does not mean that your body also needs a total holiday. It is more about getting away from the city and relaxing your mind but, at the same time, working your body, giving it a regular once-a-week day of complete rest. I am sure that you do not want to come back from your holiday with a lot of weight gain and regret. If you are not careful, all the hard work you did to get into decent shape for your holiday will be wasted because of the things you did or didn't do while *on* holiday. First, you do not want all your pre-holiday effort to go down the drain. And second, you also want to be able to eat a little bit of junk food while on holiday. So exercise so that you can stay in shape and still eat a little unhealthy food—*only* if you really have to. And considering that it is not too difficult to follow a simple routine, why waste all the effort you had put in?

Yes, it is important to exercise, and it is equally important to follow a decent diet when you are out of town. Most places will have salad bars, healthy sandwiches, wholewheat pastas and delicious soups. You can sample the local junk food and eat a slice of that pizza, but balance it out with healthy meals and a good workout. Just don't have two bad meals on the same day. If you eat a heavy lunch, avoid a heavy dinner and go for healthier options. You need your nutrition even when you are on holiday. If you are staying at a hotel, the breakfast buffet will usually consist of an amazing spread of all sorts of dishes. Have a hearty breakfast as this is what starts your day and will keep you going. Have some milk and muesli, have fruit, and if you eat eggs, you could have some boiled eggs too. Starting your day with a healthy breakfast is extremely important—whether on holiday or not. So eat well. Usually, if you eat a good, satisfying, filling breakfast, you will not be tempted to eat unhealthy food. Other than a hearty breakfast, the key is to eat small. When on holiday, I often buy some dried fruit and an easy-to-eat fruit like an apple or a banana from the local stores, and I eat it a few hours after my breakfast. So if breakfast is at 9 or 10 a.m., I eat a few walnuts at 11 a.m. or noon, and lunch by 1 or 2 p.m. Then, after 2–3 hours, I usually have a fruit. Often, in the evening, I'll have a vegetable juice like carrot juice, or coconut water, followed by a nice dinner an hour or two later. This way, I feel satisfied all day and hence do not crave too much junk food. Even when out of town, try and eat something healthy. A yummy salad is always welcome, as is a great soup and, occasionally, a slice of pizza or a few fries or some other junk food—but all in limited quantities. A great evening snack is a couple of digestive biscuits, an apple or a small bottle of low-fat milk. This can be followed by a healthy dinner. Eating healthy on a holiday is quite doable—really. Try it! It is not as difficult as it sounds.

You can do so many fun activities to stay active while you are on holiday.

Coming to the very basic but extremely fun activity for most girls and women—shopping. Shopping is awesome when you are not in your city! Finding things that hopefully no one else in your social circle has, seeing 'what's in' in the city where you are and having full leeway to buy whatever you want are the basic advantages of shopping out of town. I can give you my example and tell you that whenever I have gone abroad to some shopping destination, I have usually lost weight or at least not put on any, even though I was eating French fries, ice cream and pizza every now and then—part of the reason was that I did balance it with healthy meals. I will tell you about certain places I really enjoyed shopping in. First on my list is London. Think of anything you need and I am pretty sure you will find it there. London is very easy to commute in, and the famous Oxford Street is a great place to shop at. There are hundreds of shops on that stretch to go crazy over, and when you need a break, you just need to walk a little farther to Hyde Park, park yourself in the cafe next to the lovely lake and enjoy a soup, salad or healthy sandwich. This place is a sheer treat. Another place I thoroughly enjoy shopping in is Bangkok. You should avoid brand shopping here and go look at their local markets. They are not expensive, and they have great stuff—dresses, tops and beachwear. You really have to walk to find stuff you like here, and hunting through the endless options is real fun. Other places that are great for shopping are New York, Singapore, Paris and Dubai. All these destinations are great to visit as not only do they offer fabulous shopping but also other cool activities. And being a tourist in any part of the world usually translates to a lot of walking and exploring. Museums involve much walking and can give you a good appetite for your lunch, the parks are lush and beckon to you to walk through them; walking around the city is also a must as it is often the best way to take in the local sights and sounds.

Another great holiday, which I think most teenagers and young adults would like to experience, is going to a music festival. Music festivals are gaining popularity around the world. There are different kinds of music festivals which are massive and widespread. They usually have several stages, which means you can go and listen to artistes at different arenas and enjoy the ambience of various settings. For music lovers and for all those who love dancing, this is a real treat. If you are at a music festival, it naturally means that you are going to dance and be on your feet almost all day. The sheer size of these festivals means you will have to walk a lot. One has to walk to and from the festival and, of course, move from stage to stage inside the festival. If you are at a music festival, it is nearly impossible to not dance. Dancing definitely burns a lot of calories, and I am pretty sure that the music festival sort of dancing would involve a lot of jumping, which means even more calorie burning. A little warning though: I always say that you should live life to the fullest, but you've got to be careful at these festivals. Simple things you should observe for your own safety are: buying your own drinks, not doing any drugs and exiting the scene if you feel there is a hint of drug-taking around where you are. You know when something feels fishy, you know what is right and wrong. So have a blast, but stay safe. Talking from experience, and being a teetotaller, I have had a blast at music festivals without resorting to alcohol, cigarettes or drugs. It is possible to have a great time without getting high on different substances. The music alone can get you high. All I can say is: Have fun, but don't overdo anything. Some great music festivals you could explore are Tomorrowland, Ultra Music Festival, Electric Daisy Carnival, Stereosonic and Coachella.

You can—and should—have a holiday adventure every once in a while. A holiday does not only mean lazing around and sipping a delicious drink, it can also mean a trip to the mountains, hiking and trekking. For all the extreme adventurers and daredevils out there, you could go on an adventure trip and learn skydiving or scuba diving. While learning skydiving, you could do the accelerated free-fall course or just do a tandem dive. The adrenalin rush and thrill of jumping out of a plane is something you should try and experience at least once. Australia, New Zealand, Nepal, Spain, Dubai and Russia are great places to skydive in. I went skydiving in Dubai, and it is definitely one of the most amazing and thrilling experiences of my life. The beautiful feeling of just falling freely is magical, and the view from up there is breathtaking. I can't even put into words how it felt the second I jumped out of the plane—it was just unbelievably exhilarating. I think it is a feeling everyone should experience. I loved it so much I hope to do the accelerated free-fall course soon.

I recently went on a scuba-diving trip to the Andaman and Nicobar Islands. This place is heaven on earth. I went with four of my girlfriends to Havelock Island in the Andamans to learn scuba diving.

Let me start with the first thing that got us excited. While landing at Port Blair, we saw a few islands from the plane. The view was breathtaking; all we could see were lush green islands and the clear, blue sea. That was the moment we knew that this trip was going to be one that we would never forget.

From Port Blair we had to take a ferry to Havelock, and due to our flight timings, we had to take the government-run ferry. I will be honest and tell you that the facilities on the ferry were not excellent, but it was only a 2-hour journey and hence it was manageable. What my friends and I did was get out of the seating area on to the deck of the ferry and out in the open air. That was good—really good. We sat there for over an hour and saw the islands pass by us. The pollution-free air was a delight to breathe in, and the clear water a delight to see. On reaching Havelock, we went straight to the place we were going to stay for the next eight nights. We stayed in tented cabanas, which were clean and spacious and had attached bathrooms. What was great was that there was no TV, no AC, and no 3G or 2G network, which meant no WhatsApp and Facebook. The only way people could get in touch with us was through the traditional landline. It was extremely peaceful. Our tent was a 2-minute walk from the white-sand beach, and the water was crystal clear. It was amazing to be able to see our feet even when we were in waist-deep water.

Our scuba-diving lessons started the very next day, and we had some amazing instructors. They could answer each and every question we asked and, trust me, we asked some really strange questions. They were friendly and yet got the work done. We did the Advanced Open Water Diver Course, so now I can confidently call myself an advanced scuba diver. The deepest we went was 30 metres. We did a night dive and went to 2 shipwrecks, one of which was 80 metres long and had sunk around 50 years ago. We saw a lot of underwater life and learned to appreciate it even more. The highlight was seeing jellyfish, octopuses, barracudas and eight sharks! We also saw dolphins, three of them swimming together. The small fish were splendid too, the colours ranging from neon green, blue and yellow to black and grey. Oh, and we found Nemo—quite a few Nemos, actually. We learned how to talk underwater through signs and signals, and I would like to think my friends and I even invented a few new signs that can be used underwater. We danced in the water and did somersaults. I had never felt so safe and comfortable in water before. To be honest, scuba diving feels almost like a lazy sport. It is so peaceful, and you can move at your own pace, though obviously while keeping up with your group. The only tiring thing is when you are caught in a current, or when you reach the surface and you have to get back to your boat.

Scuba diving was the main purpose of our trip, but there were a lot of things that made our trip great. First, the people were wonderful, carefree and always happy; we became good friends with quite a few folks there. The atmosphere was so pleasant, it made everyone smile and stay calm. Second, we could hear the waves and see the stars in the night. It was mesmerizing. I realized that we often forget to appreciate what nature gives us, and this trip was a good reminder of that. Also, learning to do backflips off a boat straight into the sea was super. We learned how to roll off a boat, walk off a boat, and even simply fall off a boat, all of which was excellent. Playing football on the beach was great; not worrying about getting dirty and tanned was even better. I can go on about how amazing each and every thing about this trip was. I would go back again and again; in fact, I am already trying to find the time to escape once more to this paradise.

Simply put, scuba diving is a great experience, and swimming in the sea—actually *in* the sea—is a great way to spend a holiday. First, there is plenty to see and plenty to learn. It is like being part of a fabulous new world. And second—the real purpose of my little story—is to tell you how you can burn a lot of calories even while on a fantastic, relaxing holiday! One of my friends lost 2.5 kg. I lost a kilo, and this was despite the fact that we ate really well. By well, I don't mean healthy—I mean, we ate butter naan and paneer tikka and had Nutella almost every day. But we also ate one healthy meal and a good breakfast. Considering that, 1–2.5 kg lost in a week is kind of awesome. This is definitely a must-have holiday—exciting and yet relaxing.

If you can't afford to take a lot of time off, you could take weekend holidays around your city. Find a spot around your city where you can go hiking or trekking. Hiking and trekking are similar, but not the same. The main difference between the two is that hiking consists of walking in a natural environment along paths known as hiking trails, while trekking is more challenging and does not necessarily have a predetermined path; it could consist of climbing a hill, for instance. Another difference between hiking and trekking is that hiking is more of a leisure activity and is easy and moderate-paced, while trekking is more vigorous and usually has a destination or some place you want to reach. You could find a nice place around your city for a weekend getaway that offers hiking or trekking options. Some spots in Maharashtra where you can go are Shivneri Fort, Lohagad, Kalsubai Peak, Raigad or

Sinhagad. There are many places you can go trekking which are breathtaking and worth the walk, and also result in calorie loss. You can try the Roopkund trek in Uttarakhand, the Markha Valley trek in Ladakh or the Pin Parvati Valley trek in Himachal Pradesh.

Hiking or trekking is a great way to spend a long weekend and is an excellent way to refresh your mind and enjoy the serenity of nature. You get a great full-body workout, at the end of which your mind is relaxed.

Some other great activities to do while you are on holiday include skiing, rock climbing and horse riding.

You can go skiing in India or abroad. There are plenty of excellent skiing locations in India such as at Gulmarg, Auli and Pahalgam in Kashmir. If you want to ski abroad, you can go to Switzerland or Canada and have a wonderful holiday. It is said that skiing burns up to 600 calories an hour. That's not bad at all! And usually, when you go skiing, you do not ski for just an hour; you are there for quite a few hours, trying different slopes and also trying to master the technique. Skiing gives you a good overall workout. You work your hamstrings, glutes, and inner and outer thighs. You also work your biceps and triceps when you grip the poles that help steer you around. Skiing strengthens and tones your core muscles which help you balance. Naturally, you will also engage your core muscles to stay balanced and stable.

Rock climbing is a great activity and not only tests your stamina, endurance and strength but also challenges your mind and body coordination. It increases your heart rate, which makes for a great cardio workout. It works the muscles in your arms and shoulders, strengthens the core and works the legs. Rock climbing at a moderate pace for about an hour is said to burn 400 calories.

Horse riding can be done in various parts of the world. You can go to a horse-riding camp and learn how to ride; more experienced riders can go in for a cross-country camp. Horse riding is a great cardiovascular activity and an excellent way to stay in shape. It strengthens and tones the muscles in the arms and legs. It gives great shape to the core and strengthens the back muscles to help maintain good posture while riding. Cappadocia, Masai Mara, Loire Valley and Banff National Park are some great places for horse riding.

Let me tell you a little about Hazel Keech and her routine. She may seem cute and delicate, but she is extremely adventurous and outgoing. When in town, in Mumbai, she is regular with her workouts and does Pilates and altitude training 2–3 times a week. Hazel had a lower-back problem for a very long time and had been in considerable pain. She started Pilates in February 2013, and just 2 weeks into her training, she came to me saying her pain seemed to have vanished. Hence, goal number one was achieved quite quickly. The next goal was getting fitter and stronger and ensuring that her pain did not recur. We have been doing regular training to strengthen her core and glutes to ensure she can dance and do all the other activities she wants to do, without having to worry about a recurrence of the pain. Hazel is one of the few people who religiously do their homework—just a few exercises that she does at home on the days she does not come to the studio. I give her different workouts for when she is travelling on work or when she is on a vacation. These workouts hardly take 30 minutes and are very effective and important. Also, this helps ensure that she maintains, if not necessarily loses, her weight while out of town. Hazel goes on adventure holidays. One thing she seems to enjoy a lot is surfing. She surfs often, which is a good way to stay active on holiday. Surfing is a great way to burn calories, learn something new and generally have a blast. Hazel is a great example of how to enjoy a holiday and still stay in shape.

Make sure you follow all the safety procedures when trying out any adventure activity, and do it only in safe places with professionals.

Now, let us move on from adventurous activities to the more traditional ways of working out. If you are on holiday and are staying at a hotel, you would most likely have access to a gym or a swimming pool. Utilize these services. Go for a 20-minute jog on the treadmill or do some laps in the pool. The gym will have weights—use some of them. A sample/simple workout would be to do a 5-minute slow walk on the treadmill as a warm-up, and then increase your speed to a jog or a run. You could either stay at a constant pace for 10–15 minutes, or do interval training, where you run for one minute, then walk briskly for another minute up to 10–15 minutes, and then slow down and walk for another 2–5 minutes to cool down. You could use free weights after this. Start with bicep curls, triceps, then overhead press and lateral raises—do 10–15 repetitions to work the arms. You could do 3 sets of each. Also, add some abdominal work and do 20 crunches, 20 repetitions of obliques and 20 sit-ups. If time permits, you could also do a few squats and lunges and, voila!—in less than 30 minutes, you have managed a pretty good workout.

In case you do not have access to a gym, you can practise the following routines in your room. No excuses for not working out, you see!

❖ **Tricep Dips:** Do 20 repetitions. Place your palms on the bed, and your legs on the floor in front of you. Lower your body slowly towards the floor until your elbows are at about 90 degrees and then press up. Ensure that your shoulders stay relaxed throughout. Keep your core engaged while breathing in on the way down and breathing out as you press up.

❖ **Push-ups:** There are 3 ways you can do a push-up, depending on your strength level. The easiest is placing your palms against the wall, a little lower than shoulder level. It is okay to start like this. Walk away from the wall, keeping your body in a straight line from head to toe. Slowly lean towards the wall while inhaling, and then exhale, pressing into your palms to push your body back up. The second way of doing a push-up is on your knees, palms on the floor. Again, ensure you stay long in this position. Do not sink into your back and keep your core engaged. Lower your body very slowly towards the mat, bending at the elbows (make sure you do not keep your bottom up). Exhale and press into your hands to push up. The third kind of push-up is the full push-up: knees off the floor and legs straight so they can be either adducted or abducted, hip-distance apart. Ensure that your body is in a straight line from head to toe; there should be no pressure on your lower back. Inhale to lower your body down towards the mat and exhale to push it up. The slower you go, the harder it gets. Whichever way you decide to do the push-up, do at least 20 repetitions. Start slow and build it up.

❖ **Ab Prep:** Lie on a mat, keeping your back in a neutral position, following the natural curve of your spine. Do not sink into the mat. Keep your legs hip-distance apart and knees bent. Place your hands behind your head, gently supporting your neck. Inhale to stay down. Exhale and slowly lift your upper body off the mat, as though you were squeezing a pencil under your chest. Inhale to lower your body back on to the mat. Do 20 repetitions and then stay up on your last repetition and do 20 pulses (this is where you stay up and only move very little to keep squeezing that pencil).

❖ **Obliques:** The starting position is the same as the ab prep. Inhale to lift your upper thorax off the mat. Exhale to turn your upper thorax to one side, keeping your shoulders open and thinking about reaching your ribcage to the opposite knee, then inhale to the centre and exhale to the other side. Do 20 repetitions.

❖ **Toe Touch:** Start with your legs in a tabletop position, knees flexed and feet off the floor with your calves parallel to the floor. Your head and shoulders should be relaxed and your palms should be resting beside you. Slowly exhale to lower one leg towards the floor and, without changing the angle of your knee, lower it by taking it away from the hip joint, and touch the toe to the floor and then inhale to lift it up. Repeat with the other leg. Alternate the legs for 20 repetitions. Ensure that there is no tension in your shoulders and neck and that your back is in a neutral position and does not rock.

❖ **Oblique Can-Cans:** Begin in the same starting position as the toe touch. Slowly turn your torso to drop your legs to one side, keeping your knees together throughout, and then bring them back to the centre. Repeat on the other side. Ensure that the opposite shoulder does not come off the mat. Go as low as core engagement can be maintained. Do 20 repetitions.

❖ **Hip Rolls:** Lie on a mat, keeping your feet hip-distance apart. By 'hip distance' I mean your feet should be 'sit bones' distance apart. Keep your hands by your sides and relax your shoulders and neck. Now inhale to prepare and exhale to slowly roll off the mat and starting with your tail bone, go one vertebra at a time, all the way up to your thoracic spine. Ensure there is no weight on the neck. Inhale to stay up, keeping your glutes engaged and then exhale to slowly roll down, starting with your thoracic all the way down to your neutral position. Do 5 slow, relaxed repetitions, and on the sixth repetition, stay up and do 10 pulses. After you exhale to roll up, inhale to lower your pelvis just an inch or two and then exhale to go back up, keeping your glutes squeezed throughout, up to 10 pulses and then inhale to stay and exhale to roll down.

❖ **Side-lying Lifts:** Lie down on one side, ensuring that your body is in a straight line from head to toe. Your hips should be stacked and head relaxed on the lower arm—not the palm as this changes the alignment and causes undue tension on the wrist. Ensure that your core is engaged and you are not sinking into the mat.

- *Straight up*: Slowly lift the top leg, keeping your core engaged and glutes squeezed, and then lower it. Go slow, it's not about taking it higher. It is more important to keep your core engaged and glutes squeezed to avoid falling forward or back. Do 10–20 repetitions.

- *Circle*: Remember that your body is the centre of the circle. So rotate your leg forward only as much as you can take it back. Start one way and then the other. Do 10 repetitions each way.

- *Lift both Legs*: Keep your feet together. Exhale and lift both your legs together and inhale to lower them. Do 20 repetitions.

Don't forget to do the full set on the other side.

❖ **Arm Circles:** This is simple but effective. Stand straight. Lift your hands up and to the side and keep them at shoulder level. Do 20 circles one way and then 20 the other way, moving from the shoulder joint. Once this becomes easy, you can increase the repetitions even to 50 each way.

❖ **Squats:** Stand with your feet slightly more apart than hip-distance, and pointing slightly outwards. The weight of your body should be towards your heels and on the balls of your feet. Your toes should be able to wiggle during the entire movement. Look straight ahead and not down towards the floor. Hold your hands straight out, parallel to the floor and your spine in a neutral position. Now, inhale to lower your body by pushing your hips out towards the back, ensuring that your knees do not turn inwards; they should be over your feet through the entire exercise. Try and go low enough, so that your hip joint is parallel to the floor. Then exhale, press into your heels and keep the balls of your feet on the floor too, to straighten your knees. Keep your glutes squeezed and ensure that your back is in a neutral alignment throughout and that there is no unnecessary rounding or extension of your spine. Do 20–30 repetitions.

- ❖ **Lunges:** Make sure your upper body is straight, shoulders relaxed and spine in neutral alignment. Pick a spot in front of you and look straight at it so that you don't keep looking down while doing this exercise. Step forward with either leg and lower your hips until both your knees are bent at about a 90-degree angle. Ensure that your knees are aligned with your ankles and not turning inwards or outwards. Your front knee should not go ahead of your ankle and the back knee should not touch the ground. Then push back with your front leg, with more weight on the heels, to go back to the starting position. You can do 10–20 repetitions on each side.

- ❖ **High Knees:** Keep your body straight, feet slightly apart. Stretch your hands in front of you at about hip level. It is as if you are running in one place, lifting your knees up in front towards your palms. Ensure that you touch each leg to the hands alternately. Land soft, and try and stay on your toes to reduce the impact on the knees. You can do 3–4 sets of this with one minute on and a 20-second break.

Even the Tabata interval, spoken about earlier, can be done. In just 4 minutes, you will end up working hard and burning calories.

These are just a few exercises you can do in your room, but they are very effective and work all the major muscle groups. They will keep your fitness level up while you are on holiday. You can always play around with the number of repetitions and the sets you do to ensure the workout is good for your fitness level. No matter how fit you are, these exercises, if done correctly and with the ideal number of repetitions, will give you a good workout.

You can even do cardiovascular exercises in your room. For example, the high-knee exercise works the legs while burning calories; the other exercises you can do are jumping jacks, burpees and mountain-climbers. All these exercises thoroughly work the legs, arms and core while burning some serious calories. Carry your skipping rope when you go on holiday. A skipping rope is a great investment; it can give you an amazing workout and is also easy to carry. If you have place in your room or any other open space, skipping is a wonderful cardio exercise. It is super effective, tones your legs, works your arms and makes you burn a lot of calories. Even 10 minutes of skipping is a great workout. So to put it simply, no matter where you are in the world, which hotel you are staying at, or what facilities are available, you can always do an effective workout.

A holiday can be exciting, thrilling, adventurous and relaxing, but you can still stay in shape and maintain your weight, coming back from your holiday not only relaxed and happier but also fitter and stronger. All I can say is: Don't stop! Just keep moving.

ACKNOWLEDGEMENTS

I wish to start by thanking my parents for believing in me, supporting me and always having faith in me. Without them, I would be nothing. Thanks to their confidence and faith in me, I have been able to achieve whatever I have. I also wish to thank my mother for patiently reading everything I wrote and guiding me, giving me her valuable inputs and helping me through it all. I wish to thank my dad, who has shared his complete knowledge of fitness with me—it is due to him that I love fitness so much and have made it such a major part of my life. Their motivation has kept me going.

I wish to thank the love of my life, my little pug, Choco. Although he cannot exactly give me inputs, his constant company by my side as I wrote this book greatly helped me. Whenever I felt stressed, tired or discouraged, all I had to do was pet him and play with him, and my thoughts would suddenly be clear again.

I thank the entire team at Random House for believing in me and giving shape to my ideas in the form of this book. I especially wish to thank the editors who got me going and helped me make this book what it is today. It is their constant guidance and their patience that has made this happen. They have guided me throughout this journey. Trisha Bora, Pallavi Narayan, Rachita Raj and Milee Ashwarya have all been an extremely important part of this journey.

A big thank you to my Nani and Nana for their constant encouragement and love, without which nothing would be possible. My heartfelt thanks also to my Dada and Dadi for their support and guidance.

Thanks to my friends who were as excited as I was when they learned I was writing this book. Their enthusiasm and spirit have helped me immensely, and they all have, in their own way, guided me and taught me things throughout my journey. Their unconditional love and faith in me has made me what I am today.

My thanks to Lisa Haydon, who started out as a client, but who has now become a dear friend. Her positivity and love have been extremely motivating. She truly does spread happiness wherever she goes. I thank her for taking out time from her busy schedule to write the Foreword for my book.

Many thanks to Manasi Scott, who has been there for me all through the way and guided me like an elder sister. She is the sister I never had.

Thanks to my *foi* (aunt), Swaroop Sampat Rawal, for showering me with love and being a true inspiration.

I am indebted to my entire family for their encouragement, love and support.

And, finally, I wish to thank my wonderful clients, who have been extremely supportive and have also given me their valuable inputs throughout this journey. Their notes, tips and experiences have been of great help. I really do think I have been blessed with the best clients ever. They have been extremely considerate and loving and have thus helped me write this book.

A NOTE ON THE AUTHOR

At just twenty-one years of age, Namrata Purohit is fitness coach to some of the best-known faces in the Indian fashion, film and sport industries. She loves life and aspires to get people fit the healthy and fun way.

A certified Pilates instructor, Namrata started her career at the age of sixteen, and is one of the youngest trained Stott Pilates instructors in the world. She runs her own fitness studio, The Pilates and Altitude Training Studio (www.pilatesaltitude.com), which enjoys the distinction of being the first studio in the world to offer both Pilates as well as a simulated altitude-training room under one roof, and which has been the Official Fitness Expert for The Femina Miss India International pageant from 2011 onwards.

Namrata has played squash and football at the national and state levels, respectively. She is also pursuing her studies and has just graduated with a major in economics. Namrata and her father, renowned fitness expert, Samir Purohit, are the official Pilates coaches to the Mumbai City FC Team 2014, a part of the Indian Super League. She lives in Mumbai.

A NOTE ON THE TYPE

Bembo is the name given to a 20th-century revival of an old-style serif or humanist typeface cut by Francesco Griffo around 1495. It is named for the poet Pietro Bembo, an edition of whose writing recorded its first instance of usage.

The typeface Bembo seen today is a revival designed under the direction of Stanley Morison for the Monotype Corporation in 1929.

Bembo is a good choice for expressing classic beauty or formal tradition in typographical design. It has been noted by the authors of *Typographic Specimens: The Great Typefaces* for its ability to 'provide a text that is extremely consistent in colour and texture . . . [enabling it to] remain one of the most popular book types since its release'.